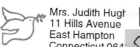
"I was only half way through my own chemotherapy treatment when I received the page proofs of *Wrestling with God and Cancer.* It was just what I needed—a long conversation over a backyard fence. Beverly Lancour Sinke is a woman of deep faith. She not only accepts suffering but regards it as holy. This is not just a book for cancer victims. She teaches all of us that we can live our lives in light rather than in darkness."

Tim Unsworth
Columnist, *National Catholic Reporter*

"I was deeply moved by this manuscript. Dr. Sinke is, first of all, a very good storyteller, and her integration of her personal story with the 'ultimate questions' is very effective. This format allows the reader to make his/her own personal connections with the story, and consequently with the 'questions' it raises in a way that is meaningful and powerful."

Margaret Stack, Ph.D.
Director of Clinical Psychology Training
University of Detroit Mercy
Detroit, MI

"*Wrestling with God and Cancer* made me wonder, laugh, and cry. Beverly Sinke balances thought-provoking reflection from her training as a theologian with moving personal confession from her never-ending battle with cancer to leave you overwhelmed by her courage, honesty, and above all her faith."

V. James Mannoia, Jr.
President, Greenville College
Greenville, IL

"Although I have never met Beverly Lancour Sinke, I now feel that I know her well. Her story provides eloquent testimony to how suffering can make us strong and doubt can inspire deeper, truer faith. I am especially thankful for Beverly's honesty and vulnerability. Her book will sow intellectual and spiritual seeds in many lives that will bear fruit for years to come."

Evan Drake Howard
Author, *Suffering Loss, Seeking Healing*

"Confronted with doubts, fears, certitudes, and awe, Beverly Sinke sets forth in a down-to-earth manner how she was grasped by God, held by family and friends, and drawn to the Ineffable."

Josephine A. Gaugier, O.P.
Director of Lay Ministry Formation
Diocese of Saginaw, MI

"This book is a challenge that engages the inner self when confronted with the crises of our human condition. It demonstrates the power of the mind and spirit to overcome in the face of suffering and pain."

V. James Mannoia, Ph.D.
Wilmore, KY

"Beverly Sinke brings together here a stirring account of crises she has experienced in her life, her reflections on those through the years, spiritual reading that has both sustained her and helped her to make sense of them, and her hard-won integration of all of this. While her style invites us to read on simply to find out what happened to her, she taps into the universality so that we recognize the richness of her sensemaking for us as well."

Margot Hover, D.Min.
Teaching Chaplain, Memorial Sloan-Kettering Cancer Center
New York, NY

"Anyone who has 'experienced' life can easily find herself or himself within the pages of this book. It is a powerful reminder to all who read it of the movement of God within the life of the human person. Beverly Sinke is remarkable in her ability to draw the reader into her own unique journey with God."

Dr. Anneliese Sinnott, O.P.
Vice President for Academic Affairs and Dean
Ecumenical Theological Seminary

For more testimonials turn to page 85

BEVERLY LANCOUR SINKE, PH.D.

# WRESTLING
## *with* GOD *and*
# CANCER

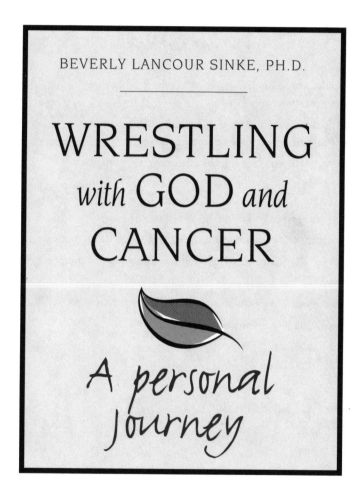

*A personal Journey*

TWENTY-THIRD PUBLICATIONS
BAYARD Mystic, CT 06355

# Acknowledgments

My thanks to my family and friends who read my book
and gave me their support.

Special thanks to: Fr. Anthony Kosnik whose unrelenting belief
in me brought this book to completion;

Sr. Donna Hart who first suggested I write about my struggle
with cancer;

Dr. and Mrs. James Mannoia who critiqued my work
and encouraged me to publish;

my daughter-in-law, Laura, who read and retyped my manuscript;

my niece, Lori Lancour, who aided me in my part of the publishing tasks;

and Twenty-Third Publications and the people I worked with
there who made a dream become a reality.

Twenty-Third Publications/Bayard
185 Willow Street
P.O. Box 180
Mystic, CT 06355
(860) 536-2611
(800) 321-0411

ISBN: 0-89622-998-X
Library of Congress Catalog Card Number: 99-75665
Printed in the U.S.A.

# Dedication

To my husband, Robert,
whose freeing love
releases me to follow my bliss


To my family, the catalyst for writing this book

My children:
Ray and Laura, Chad and Debby, Greg and Kerry,
Aaron and Cari
My grandchildren already here:
Miranda, Matthew, Kaitlynn, and Cassandra
And the grandchildren to come...

# Table of Contents

# Foreword

The story you are about to read is the story of the journey of a soul wrestling to give honest expression to a lifelong struggle with the ultimate questions. What really is life all about? Who is God? Where is God in all of this—particularly in the tragedies and losses of life? What is the role of prayer? How ought we to pray?

But this is not an abstract, theoretical exploration of these questions. It arises out of the real-life experience and the lifelong struggle of the author. As a wife, a mother, a layperson, Bev Sinke writes with a clarity, simplicity, and concreteness that enables readers to appreciate and enter more deeply into the mystery she is attempting to describe. As a serious scholar well versed in the philosophical, psychological, and theological sciences, she deftly weaves the insights of experts in these fields to add depth and confirmation to her personal experience.

The beauty of this work is that it gives expression to life experiences that are common enough to many but seldom appreciated for their true worth. It will help others to recognize the presence of God in places and events—even in the tragedies. In recounting her own developing efforts at prayer, Bev helps readers to identify and perhaps be introduced to new ways and new forms of welcoming and encountering the "Ineffable." Her twenty-year-long struggle with cancer dramatically gives witness to the off and on, up and down, roller-coaster ride of a soul struggling to stay with its God until it finally reaches Augustine's conclusion: "Restless is my soul, O God, and restless will it be until it finally rests in Thee!"

In this era when there is scarcely a family that has not been touched by the big "C" or other senseless tragedies, this alone would be well worth the price of admission. But there is so much more here to help you discover the meaning of life, to encounter the "Ineffable," and to grow in your prayer life! As one who has been privileged to be a com-

1

panion on some of this journey I reverence the courage and risk Bev took to bare her soul with such candor. This will be a special gift to other puzzled wayfarers seeking guidance on their journey to Life! Enjoy the ride!

Anthony R. Kosnik

# Introduction

To encounter mystery is to interact with the essence of life. The following three stories are about such encounters. I share them in the hope that they will encourage you in your journey. Perhaps they will help you to recognize God's presence in your times of difficulty. Perhaps they will speak to an emptiness within you that seeks fulfillment. If my stories move you to search for deeper meaning in life, they will have accomplished my goal.

I hope, too, that my stumbling and bumbling will convince you that a deep relationship with the Transcendent is possible; it is not reserved solely for professed religious. Sacramental moments *are* readily available to those of us who are deeply enmeshed in the secular world. There is no double standard in the spiritual quest.

Thomas Merton writes that we receive God's very life in direct proportion to our desire to receive. I believe that when we are open to God and put away our preconceived notions, we will be able to see God in many surprising ways and places. This openness, combined with a sincere desire, is the only component necessary for such a relationship.

Life is permeated with meaning. God is always in the process of giving. It is our challenge to become aware of God's caring presence in our lives. In so doing we will soon learn that our gracious God meets us where we are—not where we think we *should* be!

A possibility is a hint from God. One must follow it....
It is very dangerous to go into eternity with possibilities
which one has oneself prevented from becoming realities.

—SØREN KIERKEGAARD

And so I share my story...
—BEVERLY LANCOUR SINKE, PH.D.

Story One

# Wrestling with God

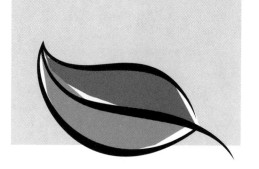

# Restlessness

*Why be concerned with meaning? Why not be content with satisfaction of desires and needs? The vital drives of food, sex, and power, as well as the mental functions aimed at satisfying them, are as characteristic of animals as they are of man. Being human is a characteristic of a being who faces the question: After satisfaction, what?*

—ABRAHAM HESCHEL

Abraham Heschel writes that the way to the holy is through the secular. With this statement he is acknowledging that the mundane day-to-day occurrences in our lives are the milieu in which God draws us. This path does not necessitate being a priest, nun, minister, or rabbi. Rather, it calls us to be active participants in the daily events that unfold in our lives. This certainly has been true in my case.

It was the middle sixties and I was knee-deep in family life. We had two healthy active boys, ages three and five. My husband had just graduated from college and had landed a job with General Motors in Milford, Michigan. Everything was going according to schedule. We, indeed, had the good life. However, even with all of this there was a vague sense of emptiness.

Everyone, I suspect, has sporadic stretches in their faith life when everything they do lacks enthusiasm. Nothing holds them captivated. The zest simply goes out of living. I know that this is simply part of the human condition. We can't always be on the mountaintop. In fact, boredom can be a gift from God. Restlessness sets in. Nothing is satisfying. One searches for meaning in life amid the tedium. Such reflective searching can lead to the ultimate questions: Who am I? Why am I here? What is my purpose? Boredom can lead to a deeper, more intense search for God.

In my case this boredom began to surface at Mass. Prayer was stale, monotonous. I could feel myself wandering farther and farther away. This attitude of apathy slipped up on me so silently. Before I realized it, I had not been to church in a month. I knew something had to be done to counteract this backsliding.

One afternoon I sat down with God and we had a heart-to-heart talk. "Now look, Lord, you have got to do something that will get me back on the straight and narrow. You're losing me." With naivete that astonishes me even today, I blithely asked for a cross that would restore my enthusiasm.

I wasn't recklessly foolish. I wasn't going to take any chances with God getting carried away. I was specific in my request. I didn't pretend to be brave. I just wanted to get a job done. I told God a very small cross would do nicely.

As I recall this past event, I realize that I was young and inexperienced in the workings of the Spirit. Today I would never dream of asking for crosses. I realize now that if we can handle with gracefulness what life brings our way, we will do well. I am not even always successful at that.

As I look back, though, this truly was a grace-filled moment even if foolish. My ultimate goal was to continue my journey toward God. Reflection, brought on by the boredom, helped me to recognize that my drive to fulfill this goal was weakening. I needed to turn the situation around. Besides, God can handle good intentions mixed with brashness. God does not demand perfect love, only the flawed love of people on their way to wholeness.

As usual, during my prayer time there was silence from the other side. However, at this stage of the journey that was all I ever expected—a me-sided monologue. Somehow, though, I always knew I had been heard. I waited for my cross.

# The Sorrow

*Man's attitude to his existence... the way in which man accepts his fate and all the suffering it entails, gives him ample opportunity to add a deeper meaning to his life.*
                                              —VIKTOR FRANKL

Can you picture my surprise the next month when I discovered I was pregnant! Our youngest, Chad, was three years old and no longer a baby. The family looked forward to the new addition. However, I thought at the time that this was a funny "cross," a baby is such a blessing. Then I began to remember that ninth-month stretch where comfort is a condition of the past and you think your time will never come. So anxious are you to bring this baby into the world, you forget the pain you went through with your last delivery.

Once the baby has arrived and the celebrating is over, the reality sets in quickly—the diapers, the bottles, the two a.m. feeding, the continuous lack of sleep, and finally, the heaviest burden of all, the awesome responsibility for another life. A baby is so dependent, but so demanding about it. I decided that in a certain way having a baby could be considered a cross. Besides, life had indeed taken on new meaning. My prayer had been answered. I closed this file and tucked it away deeply in my memory bank. I moved enthusiastically into the excitement a baby brings.

Around the second or third month of pregnancy a red flag went up. I told my husband that I sensed something was terribly wrong, but I couldn't put a name to it. There was something just not right. I had carried two other children so I knew what carrying a child was all about. It was nothing I could put my hands on, nothing physical, nothing concrete. I was healthy, young, and enthusiastic about what we hoped would be our first girl. Yet, there was this nagging, vague feeling. After comforting assurances from my husband and doctor that everything must be fine for I wasn't the least bit sick, I put this thought aside and continued to make preparations for the pink nursery.

My parents lived in the Upper Peninsula. I was quite surprised then when my mother said that she would be coming two weeks before the baby was due. She said she was anxious to put the finishing touches on the nursery. We joked about positive thinking enhancing our chances for a girl. The room was painted, and pink frilly dresses hung in the closet. The family waited in anticipation for the new arrival.

The long-awaited day finally arrived and would you believe it, I had the flu. What timing! You can't tell Mother Nature to hold off, however, so I delivered a baby boy, flu and all. As soon as I held the little bundle, I knew we had a "keeper" as we say in our family. We still had another chair to fill, we had wanted at least four children. Our next baby would be the girl. Life was moving right along on schedule.

Terry, our son, was kept in isolation away from the other babies. The mother had delivered with the flu, the baby had the flu. It was a natural conclusion. Problems set in with feeding immediately. The baby required extra attention. No serious problem I was told, just extra care and special bottles. I could go home, but Terry would stay a few extra days to get a good start on life. The nurses were still having some difficulty getting him to drink the milk. He seemed to have no strength left after taking a couple of ounces. He just needed to gain a little weight, get a little stronger. I could come back in a couple of days and take him home. I would need the extra rest to care for Terry who needed to eat every two hours.

It sounded like a good idea. I went home to rest for a couple of days before taking on the responsibility for another life. What started out as a very restful day would end up sapping the very life force out of me and strain to the breaking point my relationship with my God.

I remember vividly, even today, the phone call that came that very evening. "Come to the hospital immediately, your baby is in very serious trouble." "Is there anything you can do?" I asked. My doctor's voice was strangely subdued, "We have done everything possible." I quickly replied, not wanting to waste precious moments, "Then rush the baby to the University Hospital in Ann Arbor." I had delivered at a small but competent hospital. Ann Arbor, however, had all the latest technology. I did not want them to wait for Bob and me before they transferred Terry. We could meet them at the University Hospital.

The tone of his voice should have told me there was something more. But one is never prepared for the news I was about to hear. There was silence and then softly my doctor said: "Your baby has already died." He didn't want to tell me over the phone, but when I insisted certain steps be taken immediately, he had no other choice.

It is odd what one remembers. I have often wondered why certain memories come to mind while others are hidden away forever. I don't remember what I said to Bob when I hung up the phone. I don't remember what I told my mom and the boys when we left. I don't even remember the conversation that took place on that cold November night in the half-hour drive to the hospital. I do remember the television movie we were watching, "Stalag 17," starring William Holden. Why would I remember that particular fact? Selective memory at work never fails to amaze me. We are such complex creatures! I'm sure the other memories were just too painful, and so I buried them deeper, out of reach.

We arrived at the hospital around ten p.m. and went immediately to the maternity ward. The ghostly quiet and dimly lit hallways added to our eerie situation. No one was in sight. We looked around and noticed a bassinet at the other end of the hall. We walked over and inside was our dead baby boy. I didn't cry. I don't remember feeling anything. I was in shock. At this point the mind took control, the body had shut down.

Being the cradle Catholic that I was, the first thought that came to mind was baptism. We must save our baby from Limbo! So there in that darkened hall I took spittle and baptized my baby, harboring the secret hope that Terry had not been dead too long so the baptism would "take." Twenty-five years ago Limbo was that theological construct where unbaptized babies spent eternity. They weren't bad, so they shouldn't go to hell, but neither were they baptized, so they couldn't go to heaven. They went to Limbo. It made perfect sense in a black-and-white theological mindset. In the Pre-Vatican II church you knew what the rules were and you followed them to the letter. I knew what I had to do, so I baptized my dead child.

As I write out this scenario some twenty-five years of life experience later, I am appalled at the scene I recall. How awful that these young broken-hearted parents felt they had to baptize their dead baby to save it from an eternity away from God. Where was God's love? God's mercy? Even God's justice? A baby is innocence personified. I am just grateful that my concept of God today has deepened. Yesterday's stern legalistic judge has become for me today a God of unconditional love, a God who accepts and affirms people who are in the process of becoming.

The doctor was truly puzzled over why the baby had suddenly died, so we agreed to an autopsy. The results showed the baby had a hole in the heart. Years of surgery would have been required, had they been able to save him. The flu symptoms had masked the real problem. The doctor assured us that the heart was so badly damaged that there was really nothing we could have done. This problem with the heart occurred early in the pregnancy. As the doctor continued to explain how the heart was formed, my mind immediately shot back to that sense of uneasiness I had experienced.

To this day I am not exactly sure what to make of this experience. The timing of the two events, the malformation of the heart and my sense of danger, was uncanny. Is the intimate connection between mother and baby so one that I would somehow know something was wrong? This sensing of danger was also picked up by someone else. It was only after the baby had died that mom told me the real reason she had come early. She confided that one day while she was praying she sensed a cloud descending over the family. She could not tell who it concerned exactly, only that it was my family. The feeling was so strong that she wanted to come immediately to be near us.

I sensed the danger; my mother sensed the danger. I can't explain how. It doesn't happen often, this sensing, but when it does it puts me in touch with the mystery of life. This mystery, which is the underpinning of all reality, is more than what can be seen, touched, measured, or weighed. My experience confirms this. At times the veil is pulled back slightly and we are given brief access to this realm of mystery.

# The Struggle

*Astonishing and stately is our soul—the place where the Lord dwells. Therefore God wants us to respond whenever we are touched, rejoicing more in God's complete love than sorrowing over our frequent failings.*

*—JULIAN OF NORWICH*

Parents should never have to bury a child. That is not the natural order of things. When it does happen it reveals clearly the disorder in the world. The tragedy touched all of us deeply. I saw my stoic husband cut to the very core, "I didn't even get to hold my son." I simply gave myself permission to cry anywhere and anytime. But at the funeral a question from Ray, my five-year old, was one that would continue to haunt me. It kept ringing in my ear, "Mommy, why did God take him? I didn't even get to see my little brother."

As the grieving process took hold, rumblings began to bubble up from the depths of me. I echoed my son's question—why, why did God take our baby? Did I do something wrong? Was God trying to teach me a lesson? Was God testing my faith? If that was the case, I didn't think that was a fair way of doing it. I didn't deserve this treatment.

I put the questioning aside for awhile, hoping it would lose some of its force. It not only did not go away but returned more powerful than before. Didn't God know how much this hurt? What kind of God did I serve that had this pain-filled plan for me? Did God ever really care? If I were God, I wouldn't treat my people this way.

This was the first time I had experienced such rebellion. I simply could not square my image of God with the suffering I was going through. My image was a God who had power over my life, who had a master plan for me, who cared for me. People said this was God's will and I should accept it as such. That simply did not make sense. They wanted me to believe a God of love was the source of this pain! Well, I made up my mind that I wanted no part of this God.

Why didn't I simply ignore the questions that kept coming to the surface? Maybe that works for some people, but it is not my way. I didn't particularly like thinking about my God in this way. I didn't want to harbor doubts and ill-will. God and I had had some good times together in the past. As in any honest relationship, we didn't always see eye to eye on everything, but eventually I would come around to God's way of thinking. We had worked out our differences before, and I felt that we would do it again.

Besides, why should I hide my questions this time? God was always big enough in the past to handle them. I felt it was intellectually dishonest to deny their existence. Furthermore, if God and I didn't work it through, it would be a surrender imposed from without rather than coming from within. It would be a surrender I couldn't "own." That type of acceptance would never have been permanent for me, for it wasn't rooted deeply enough in my being.

In the past I just had to pray and struggle with difficulties and the insight would finally come. This time it was different. No insight was forthcoming. The struggle continued. I had heard all my life about this God who loved us so much, a stern God, yes, but not uncaring. If you followed the rules, God came through for you. I did not understand. I had kept my part of the bargain. God was failing me!

Up until then, when the events in my life were meaningful I had had no trouble buying into God's plan for me. I just did not know how God figured into the picture when such meaningless suffering entered my life. I know that we can't go through life without pain and struggle, but before it had not been senseless pain. Who benefited from the loss of our baby? My experience critiqued my concept of God, and God came up wanting!

This questioning process went on for about eight weeks. I had tried as best I could to come out on the side of God, but the evidence came in overwhelmingly in favor of lived experience. It never entered my mind to change my *concept* of God. I resolved the problem by concluding that there simply was no God. It was all a great hoax, a comfort that allowed people to face the harsh reality of life. They blindly accepted without question this "will" of God that produced such pain. My questioning had led me to see the mockery of a God imposing suffering on unsuspecting people. I was angry and hurt. I had been duped by religion into believing in a loving God. It was all fraud. I was alone and on my own.

I did not realize at the time that I was wrestling with the question that has plagued philosophers and theologians for centuries: how do we account for evil and suffering in a world created by a loving God? However, for me it was more than an abstract issue. The meaningless death of my baby was very concrete. I struggled to make sense of it.

When a person is killed in a car accident or when people are oppressed due to racism, we can account for the evil by the choices of other people acting out of their free will. Another person has chosen to do the evil, another person is responsible for the suffering. The driver of the other car may have had too much to drink. Perhaps fear or greed is what motivates racists. These are acceptable explanations, though certainly not comforting.

However, how do we account for those other tragedies where no human choice is involved? The tornado that takes a life, the famine that results in widespread starvation? These events have no human agent. I suppose that is why traditionally people have credited God with these actions. It is more comforting at least to have some explanation for evil in life than to be at the mercy of the unknown. Erich Fromm captures this human characteristic when he writes: "People would rather have the security of false truth than the freedom of ambiguous reality" (*Man for Himself: An Inquiry into the Psychology of Ethics*). I wanted nothing to do with false truth, so I forfeited my relationship with God.

# The Caring Presence

*Awe enables us to perceive in the world intimations of the divine, to sense in small things the beginning of infinite significance, to sense the ultimate in the common and the simple; to feel in the rush of the passing the stillness of the eternal.*

—ABRAHAM HESCHEL

All the time this inner turmoil was going on, I was involved with work at church. I washed and ironed the albs and altar linens. Since the church was kept locked when services were over, this work entitled me to a key. I picked up and delivered the linens at all hours of the day. Even though I had now decided that God did not exist, I continued with this work. It would take time to find someone to replace me. I had taken on this job and I wasn't about to let my friends down. I would wait patiently until someone stepped forward to relieve me of this now meaningless chore. What happened next still raises goose bumps twenty-five years later, so strong was the impact.

One Sunday afternoon, after I had reached the conclusion that this adult was not going to be taken in by that childish story of God, I went to church to put away the altar linens. I don't remember why, but I decided to go into the church proper. I sat there before the tabernacle where I once believed Jesus was present. The longer I sat there the angrier I became. Finally I literally shook my fist and blurted out, "You don't exist. You're a fraud. I'll prove to you that you're not real. I'm going to get up and walk out of this church right now. If you're real, there will be someone at the back door." The church was locked and empty. No one was ever around late Sunday afternoon. It was a safe challenge and I knew it. I had issued my ultimatum. I would show that non-existent God!

Can you imagine my utter astonishment when I saw the pastor at the back door! He was just standing there. He had no key. He couldn't get in. He was out riding his lawn tractor, not expecting to go into the church. To say the least, I was speechless. When I let him inside he said something to the effect that he had just decided on the spur of the moment to stop in. He realized when he got to the back door that the church would be locked.

I had issued my challenge and God had answered. Where no one should have been—there now stood a priest! How did I feel? I was stunned beyond belief, relieved, thrilled, confused, ashamed, sorry, and thankful, and just about in that order.

In my hurt and anger I had lashed out at the Lord of the cosmos. Who was I to throw out such a challenge to God? The biblical Job immediately sprang to mind. Our God, the outrageous lover, stooped to my level in order to touch my heart. Love is transforming! I was totally overwhelmed when I saw the pastor standing there. I was even more amazed when he said that his visit was spontaneous. For me, this truly was a sacramental moment. God was present—in the person who stood at the back door responding to his own inspiration. People are a precious channel that God often uses to touch the hurting heart. Sometimes human beings are the only presence of God that some people ever encounter. What a responsibility this calls us to!

How do we rationally explain such experiences? Some would simply say it is a coincidence and leave it at that. Unless experience falls neatly into known categories of understanding, it is suspect and so laid aside. We must leave room for the mystery in our lives. We can touch into greater depths of understanding if we can only be open to the mystery that surrounds us. This event was dripping with meaning. It was no chance happening. It was the God of surprises at work again in my life.

Carl Jung, the Swiss psychologist, suggests that we need an interpretive principle other than cause and effect for understanding such happenings. He says that there are far too many such "coincidences" in life. Jung posits the principle of synchronicity to account for this phenomenon. The challenge to God on my part and the visit to the church by the priest were in no way connected by cause and effect. Each action originated from a different cause. With Jung's interpretive construct, these seemingly unconnected events are an integral part of this other set of laws that operate under the principle of synchronicity. The universe is far too complex for only cause and effect happenings. However, I needed no logical explanations. For me it was simply and clearly God at work in my life. This choice to recognize and accept the meaning in this event turned my life around. I was once again journeying with my God. Peace and tranquility returned even in the midst of the suffering. I know I would not be the person of faith I am today had I chosen to label this event "chance."

This was not to be the only serendipitous event in my life. Many followed. I had been going to morning Mass during the week. One day as I sat there I looked around and saw mostly older people. All of a sudden it dawned on me, "What am I doing here in the middle of the week? I should be home cleaning house, or having breakfast with a friend, or shopping. That is where I belong, not here with these old people!"

You might recall that twenty-five years ago the priest never gave a homily during a weekday Mass. You were in and out in twenty minutes. However, this particular day the priest stopped after the gospel and turned to the small gathering, "I just want to say something today. If you're sitting there thinking, 'What am I doing here?' don't worry about it. You're here because God wants you to be here." It was as if he had read my thoughts. Why did he choose that particular day to comment? Why not the day before or the day after? Chance? The comment was too laden with meaning for it to be mere chance! Mystery had reached out to me again and I accepted.

# Reflective Reasoning

*The true source of prayer is not an emotion but an insight. It is an insight into the mystery of reality, the sense of the ineffable...To pray is to take notice of the wonder, to regain a sense of the mystery that animates all things...Prayer is our humble answer to the inconceivable surprise of living.*

—ABRAHAM HESCHEL

With hindsight I can understand somewhat how I had ended up in a downward negative spiral. The combination of an inadequate concept of God, a terrible hurt, and my questioning stance in life all played a part. However, I feel it was secrecy most of all that fueled this rebellion.

My inadequate concept of God was partly to blame. I accepted the generally held view that it was the will of God that controlled our lives. I knew nothing at the time of Abraham Heschel's concept of co-partnership with God. Today I believe that God interacts with me. God and I together are constantly creating my response to the events of my life. My talents, my historical setting, my free will, my choices coupled with prayer, are the milieu out of which "God's will" becomes clear. God's will is not some preplanned blueprint that we must discover. Rather, it is an ongoing creative process that arises from our choices and God-given circumstances. Prayer is essential for this discernment process.

The loss of a child is simply part of the human condition. It must somehow be integrated into the evil and suffering that is a reality of life. Søren Kierkegaard, the Danish philosopher, writes that it is the duty of human consciousness to understand that there are certain things that it cannot understand. Evil and suffering fall into this category. I don't know the ultimate reason for the loss of our child. I don't have answers, only a story to tell. I do know that God is present during these times. This presence is the power that sustains our hopes, encourages our spirits, and inspires our actions when dealing with such tragedies.

Furthermore, life experience has taught me that it does no good to ask "why." We have no control over the "why." That is not our proper question. It is beyond our realm of understanding. Our energies should instead be in the pursuit of the question "how?" How am I going to respond to this particular event? How can I remove the obstacles that will allow God to transform this suffering? How can I recognize the presence of God? This allows me to be a participant in the direction my life will take. The living out of the "how" calls me into co-partnership with my God. Together we co-create my response to life with all its complexity. I am convinced today that it is not the load that weighs us down, but rather how we carry it.

All those years ago, I did not talk about or share my questions and doubts with anyone. My stance was far too subjective; I needed objectivity. My relationship at this time was very vertical, strictly God and me. What I needed was horizontal input, what I needed was people.

When we bring our doubts, questions, and problems to light, and then share them with someone we respect, we will have a far more balanced perspective. I suggest strongly that if you take your spiritual journey seriously, invite a prayer partner into your life. Find someone with whom you can share the depths of your soul. This person can be your spouse or a close friend. You can also choose someone trained as a spiritual director. And there are times when someone outside the family circle will be able to give you a more objective perspective. It is a tremendous gift to have such a soul friend and if you sincerely seek it, God will provide the right person for you.

As I continued to interact with the mystery in my life over the past twenty-five years, my perspective on the "cross-sending" has deepened. A God of love does not send suffering. To think otherwise would paint God as a terribly uncaring deity. A God who loves outrageously is not a God who gives a gift of life and then yanks it back so heartlessly. No, with my present understanding, I simply list the loss of our baby under the heading "mysteries of life." It belongs in Kierkegaard's category as one of those things that is beyond our understanding.

My asking for a cross was a controlling factor on my part. I was telling God how to answer my prayer. However inadequate, it was my theological outlook at that time. But God is never stifled by our limited horizons. My underlying prayer was answered. My relationship with my God was deepened beyond my expectations.

There is no evil that cannot be transformed by the love of God. When we open ourselves to this awesome love, we are able to co-create with God our response to the evil and suffering in our life. Creating this response is our proper task, and it must include an absolute surrender to the Ineffable in our lives, to the one who is revealed as Unconditional Love. It is this act of surrender, this conviction that there is an all-caring God who will see us through all our troubles, that gives our lives meaning. And it is in this realm of meaning that we are called to live out our lives.

## Response to Story One

•What was your image of God as a child? What is your image of God today as an adult? Can you identify the experiences that helped to change/deepen your concept of God?

•Our image of God affects our prayer life. In what ways is this true for you?

•How do you understand the "will of God?" Co-partnership with God? How do you understand your participation in the "will of God?" Why is the concept of co-partnership important?

•Think of the ways you try to explain suffering in your life: will of God; evil presence; fact of life; retribution; human choice; mystery; chaos of world; other ways. Which do you tend to embrace?

•What was your response to a recent experience of unexpected loss or difficulty? Did it deepen or lessen your faith in God? Did you recognize the presence of God in the situation? What area in your life do you find it hardest to trust God? Why?

• "The transforming power of God can bring good out of evil." Can you remember a time in your life when this occurred? What were the circumstances? Was your attitude a help or a hindrance?

•What is one thing that prevents you from becoming the person you want to be? What steps can you take to eliminate the obstacles preventing this from becoming a reality?

*Let Us Pray...*

*Be joyful in hope, patient in affliction, and faithful in prayer.*
—ROMANS 12:12

My God, give me the strength, perseverance, and trust in your love to deal with the difficulties I will face in life. Help me to be open and receptive to their potential for good. I believe that they are offered possibilities for deepening my relationship with you.

I truly need the grace to recognize your presence in these difficult times. Assist me in my efforts to broaden and enlarge my own narrow view of you, the Infinite One. Allow me to see you in the variety of ways you reveal yourself. And Lord, help me to accept these graced revelations without fear.

May I be given the vision and power to pursue the unknown path, trusting in your unfailing love and never-ending mercy. And may the way I walk this path give witness to your love for your people. Amen.

Story Two

# An Awesome Interlude

# Prayer Time

Time truly does heal all hurts. In 1969 we had our baby girl, Kerry. We had put the tragedy of the past behind us. The three children were now in school and the family had settled into a comfortable routine. Morning Mass had become part of my daily schedule. Then in 1974 the God of surprises made an appearance once again. We were blessed with a baby boy, Aaron. I always harbored the secret thought that this surprise was meant somehow to make up for Terry, the baby we lost.

I soon discovered that with a newborn baby I was homebound once again. I missed going to morning Mass. I decided if I couldn't be there in body, I would be there in spirit at least. Even the baby cooperated with my plan. He was up early, bathed and dressed, had his bottle and was ready to go down for his morning nap when Mass time rolled around. Everything was working out fine.

I set up a formal structure to follow so I wouldn't be distracted. I decided a book would be of help. Someone had given me Thomas à Kempis' *Imitation of Christ* and its format lent itself to what I was trying to do, stay focused. I would read a short section and reflect on what the passage was saying to me at this particular time in my life.

This reflection led to prayer. When the prayer dried up, I would go back to my book. And so it went, reading, reflecting, praying, and then back to reading, starting the cycle over again.

I had no idea that meditation was the theological name for this activity. I had no formal training; I just stumbled along and did what came to mind.

Eventually there were times when even the book I was using was too noisy. I would set it aside and just pray. And then some days even praying was too noisy and I would just sit quietly. Again, God was guiding me, and I wasn't even aware of the gift I was being given. I did not realize I was practicing what I now know to be contemplative prayer. I did what was comfortable, what seemed right for me at the time. I did not feel the call to read or pray. I felt exceedingly peaceful if I just sat quietly in the presence of God. I followed where the Spirit led. Of course I didn't realize I was following anyone!

It was during one of these very quiet days when my faith world was turned upside down. My concept of God would never again be the same.

# The Encounter

*Love is the eternal nature of God actualized in time.*
—DAVID ROBERTS

Language is terribly limiting. Whatever I write about this encounter will never do it justice. Whatever words I use will always paint an incomplete picture. The Lord of the cosmos will not be narrowed to fit into our definitions, our categories. Abraham Heschel states that God is beyond the reach of finite notions. However inadequate though, language and finite notions are what I am forced to use to share my story.

I was in a very quiet, peaceful mode. The book had been set aside and the prayers had ceased. I was just breathing in the presence of God. An indescribable peacefulness permeated my whole being.

Then it happened! Something totally outside my previous experience broke through to my consciousness. It came on me suddenly. Every fiber of my being was touched by it. Never before in my whole life had I experienced such power, such love. It transported the core of who I was to a new realm of existence. This event would eventually revolutionize my personal relationship with my God.

What is "it"? The term "God" is so commonplace, so dull, so sterile to describe what I experienced. It is tossed around so casually.

Today I would use Heschel's term and call "it" the Ineffable, the Incomprehensible Mystery. How else can we speak of those events in life that are totally beyond our understanding, yet inspire awe and surrender!

It was like being struck by lightning. I felt like every cell in my body was lit up, every nerve was fully, totally alive. Stand up and take notice was the message that raced throughout my whole being. The picture that comes to mind is the cartoon character who sticks her finger in a light socket and every hair on her body stands on end. My whole body was being electrified with an overabundance of love. I felt it to be a love that could not give enough of itself.

And yet, it was not like this. It wasn't an outside agent in the truest sense of the word. This overwhelming love bubbled up from the depths within me. It wasn't something that was imposed from outside. This love was somehow part and parcel of who I am. And yet, at the same time I instinctively knew it was other than I.

Again, language fails me. This love that burst forth from the core of my being with such ferocity—I knew I could not properly claim it as mine. It was what Rudolf Otto calls "an experience of the numinous" (*The Idea of the Holy*). It was sheer divinity, an encounter with the unfathomable One that commands awe and reverence. I know it sounds as if I'm speaking in riddles. I can only say it was, is, mystery.

At the time I had always pictured God as "out there," someone to whom we prayed. This experience brought out what is properly called the immanent God, the God who truly dwells within us. I was awestruck by the power and the strength of this love that originated within me. I felt I could move mountains with its power. Since then I have come across Goethe's statement: "What kind of God would it be who only pushed from without." I could so identify with that thought. God lives in me in a special way.

Carl Jung says that we are splinters of an infinite deity. Well, this splinter had just caught fire. The stoic Bev, who never even cried at funerals, was suddenly overcome with emotion. I could not hold back the tears. This was not the emotional outburst of a thought process. It was instantaneous, immediate. The influx of such an overwhelming love all at once throughout my whole being simply could not be contained. I felt I would have burst at the seams had it not overflowed.

I did not call it forth nor could I send it away. I was not in control of the situation. The generosity and graciousness of this unconditional love was far superior to anything I could have conjured up. It simply came into being of its own accord. It was as if there was a power source of some kind within and somehow I had tapped into it. However, again, I must stress that although the power source was within, the energy that sustained this power source was of another origin. Language seems to be the culprit again. It simply cannot capture the experience. Bernard Lonergan in his book *Method In Theology* expresses it better poetically when echoing Pascal he states: "The gift of God's grace is the reason of the heart that reason does not know."

I knew for certain that this outrageous love that kept bubbling up could overcome any wrong. There was no sin black enough that it could not be transformed into new life through this powerful unconditional love. No evil, no person was beyond its reach. Regardless of my sinfulness, I felt that there were absolutely no barriers between my God and me. I knew experientially that I was loved, was saved, and nothing could ever take that away. I didn't have to go and perform great deeds, accomplish great tasks. This was unconditional love. This experience of love was pure gift, freely given.

Karl Rahner says that God is incomprehensible mystery but revealed as unconditional love to which our only response can be total and absolute surrender. Of course, with a mountaintop experience such as this, one cannot surrender enough. One longs to respond. At the same time one is at a disadvantage for there is no way to respond in kind to such generosity.

I gave the only gift that was truly mine to give—my love. It did not matter if it was imperfect love, warped love. At least it was my unique gift that no other could offer. Any action in the future would be grounded in this love, this desire to respond. But somehow I intuitively knew the first gift from my side had to be me. I want to stress that it is not to my credit that I responded. When you go through something as powerful as this, you literally have no choice but to respond. You are truly grasped by God and held firmly—and you know it!

In my quiet time, as the week wore on, the initial fire smoldered, flaring up now and then. I felt I was one with everything and everyone. It was the presence of this love that made the connection to all possible. A profound peacefulness that embodies surrender alternated with this fiery, electrifying love. It was, indeed, an awesome experience.

# Doubts and Fears

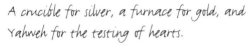

A crucible for silver, a furnace for gold, and
Yahweh for the testing of hearts.

—PROVERBS 17:3

One whole week I would step into my quiet time and this love would
bubble up from the depths. It was not as dramatic as that first day,
but still overwhelming nonetheless. There was absolutely no doubt
this love was rooted in God, was God. St. John's gospel statement,
"God is love," made perfect sense to me. God is so much more than
"God the Father." This gracious love is the sustaining reality that
keeps the world turning and the stars in place. And I was led to
understand that I was an integral part of all this through pure gift.
Abraham Heschel in *Who Is Man* writes that people are "priceless,
exceedingly precious." That captures well the atmosphere in which I
lived that week, at least in my quiet time.

It was as if I existed in two different realities. When I stepped back
into secular reality, as I now call it to distinguish it from quiet time,
I was inundated with fear and doubt. The terror I felt from the top of
my head to the soles of my feet was astonishing. The assurance and
peacefulness that were always present in quiet time were now
nowhere to be found. Doubts and questions were surfacing everywhere. These doubts and questions were almost overwhelming:
"Who do you think you are? This stuff is only for saints. God does-

n't come to sinners in this way. It is surely the devil trying to trick you."

I lived in two different realities, with one denying the existence of the other. Crossing back and forth between the two of them every day, I feared I would lose my mind. It was paralyzing. I had always been able to think things through before. Now away from my quiet time there seemed to be nothing but confusion and chaos. I kept asking myself, "Am I becoming a fanatic? Am I turning into a religious nut, the kind one reads about in the newspaper? How can old rational me be going through this? I'm always on top of things. Have I lost touch with reality?"

What seemed to confirm my fears was the fact that I knew none of my friends had had this type of experience. I was afraid that my quiet time was affecting my life adversely. Being labeled a "Jesus freak" was something to be avoided at all cost. It was okay to be religious but one stayed within certain parameters. I knew I had stepped over into a dangerous realm. We humans have a tendency to fear deeply that which we do not understand—and this was far beyond my understanding.

Why the fear and panic after such a profound encounter? I don't know. I can only relate what I went through. Maybe it explains why I share my story. If I could have laid my hands on a good book that talked about such things simply and forthrightly, as I am trying to do here, maybe I would not have had to go through all that vacillation. All I know is that the fear was strong and the doubts even stronger.

Twenty years later I realize that this was probably a very healthy process to go through. The quiet time experience was so far removed from the way I had usually experienced God. It would make sense to a rational person to question that experience. It could have been simply my check-and-balance system kicking in. How did my concept of God square with what I was going through? It didn't, so panic set in. My image of God did not fit my experience of God. And at that time I did not know one's image of God could change, could grow deeper and broader as life is lived out. Today I recognize that God constantly reveals more and more to us throughout our lifetimes. It is not God who is changing but rather our ability to understand. God reveals only as much as we are able to absorb. Today, hopefully, I am more open to the self-revealing God who is interested in my life.

Some would refer to this inward battle as Christian tension. That is far too tame a concept for what I experienced. Others would simply say it is the devil doing his job. It is the devil tempting people away from God, trying to distort the Good News. Whatever the label, it was still terrifying. Abraham Heschel says the inner universe is real. I wholeheartedly agree. The inner universe is just as motivating, just as powerful, just as beautiful as the outer universe—and at times just as terrifying.

I couldn't seem to integrate the two realities, however. As I recall this story, even I am surprised that such a powerful experience didn't automatically remove my doubts and fears. Maybe that should have been the case, but again, I can only tell my story, and that week I was literally bombarded with doubts as soon as I left my quiet time.

However, no matter the fear and panic, no matter the doubts, I simply could not resist the call to prayer. Afraid, yes, but I had to step back into my quiet time. In the end, the attraction proved to be stronger than the fear. Every day for a week this tug of war went on. It was so reassuring once I stepped over into prayer. The love would engulf me and once more I knew this realm was real and belonged to the eternal dimension.

Eventually I began to trust my experience and slowly my image of God began to take new form. The doubts and fears began to recede. They were not completely gone for I was still afraid to tell anyone what was going on. I did not want to be labeled a religious fanatic. I would keep my secret and my good reputation.

I was gradually led to understand that I wasn't losing touch with reality. I had simply discovered a deeper realm of existence. I came to realize this was God at work in my life. I had discovered Heschel's "universe within," and it was, indeed, profoundly real. This inner universe is just waiting to be discovered by any who are searching for deeper meaning in their lives.

Even after I had resolved that this experience was God interacting in my life, I still was not completely free. I was so afraid someone would catch me in my quiet time when I knew the tears would come. I came up with an imaginative solution to conceal everything. I kept an onion, half peeled, on the kitchen counter. If the doorbell rang, I could reach for my onion and account for my watery eyes. I can look back now and laugh, but then it was no laughing matter. It was done with such earnestness because I had an overriding fear of being discovered, of being labeled a fanatic.

I am amazed and amused when I recall the "onion solution." God must have been royally entertained with my antics. In time I have come to see that we serve a God who has a tremendous sense of humor. I have learned over time that the ability to laugh at oneself must be part of the spiritual journey. Anyone who considers himself/herself religious and does not have a sense of humor is missing a key ingredient of the spiritual life.

If in the future I ever decided to share this gift with others, I wanted to be able to articulate it accurately. I wanted to be able to do it justice. I also wanted, at that time, to understand it better myself. Eventually this led to college and an even deeper appreciation of what I had been given. God used my husband Bob to encourage me in this direction. When I complained that it would take me five years to get my degree and by that time I would be forty, Bob responded jokingly, "Honey, in five years you are going to be forty with or without your degree." That moved me to action. In the fall I enrolled in college and was on my way.

I want to stress that my personal encounter is not the only way to experience God. Nor is it even necessarily the best way. It is simply one way. Our God is far too creative to be limited in how to interact in people's lives. We need only be open in our searching and God will be revealed in surprising ways.

Eventually I also learned that these consolations, as I now know them to be called, were merely the frosting on the cake. The intense love and gift of tears were given to get my attention. And it certainly worked. However, there is a danger in such powerful gifts. I initially had made the mistake of being caught up in the gift rather than the giver. I was a beginner and didn't know any better. Thankfully, I was able to move forward, I am sure, due to the gracious forgiveness and abundant grace that have always accompanied me throughout my life.

# The Gifts

*How many wonders you have done for us, Yahweh our God!*
—PSALM 40:5

After this awesome encounter, I desperately needed to talk to someone about what I had been through. However, the fear was still too strong to allow me to share. It was at this time that I began to keep a journal. I did this out of necessity. I could unload, even if it was to a book that couldn't answer back, but neither would that book reveal my secrets.

The keeping of a journal enabled me to further appreciate the awesome encounter I had experienced. Later I also discovered that recording what I have been through helps me to more clearly understand the gifts I am given. The review of the year further aids me in recognizing God's presence during times of difficulty—which I otherwise might have missed.

I did not realize that the keeping of a journal was a form of prayer until I picked up Thomas Merton's *Seeds of Contemplation* where he writes: "Learn to write as a form of meditation." Once again I had evidence of the Spirit guiding my life. At that time I also recorded in my journal an entry that centered on "embarrassment about talking to a book and doubts as to the value of continuing with this technique." However, as I continued to read Merton, these questions were laid to rest. Whenever my resolve regarding the keeping of a journal and the development of the inner universe wavered, another encouraging sign was always sent my way.

Through his books, Thomas Merton became a spiritual guide for me. He always provided me with fresh insights. His ideas were stimulating and opened up exciting new paths for me to explore. He invited me to grow: "A God who remains immobile within the focus of my own vision is hardly ever a trace of the true God's passing." I learned much under his tutelage. In time my vision of God broadened tremendously.

Later on in my journey when the need arose, a soul friend was another gift I was given. The need for this gift surfaced in my journey when the mountaintop experience had passed and my prayer life became dull and dry. After the awesome encounter I had experienced, closeness to God was extremely important to me. I had truly experienced God's presence. When the time came for weaning me away from this gift, it was painful and lonely. The entry I found in my journal from that time described my feelings: "Yes, God has wined me and dined me until I was wrapped around his little finger and now he is off after someone else." I truly felt deserted. However, God always provides, and I somehow stumbled onto a spiritual director.

It was he who shored up my sagging intentions and assured me that God was still alive and very active in my life. The dryness of prayer I was experiencing was simply part of the spiritual journey. He assured me that this aridity would clarify whether I was seeking the "warm fuzzies" or God. With the encouragement of this soul friend I resolved to continue my spiritual quest.

I made the decision to meet on a regular basis with my spiritual director. I felt that my decision was affirmed when I came across this quote from Rusty Berkus: "There comes that mysterious meeting in life, when someone acknowledges who we are and what we can be, igniting the circuits of our highest potential. I see this as the appearance of an angel, and know it to be a moment of grace." If I have questions today, I have someone with whom I can discuss them, a person outside the family circle who can be objective and who (unlike my journal), can talk back.

This awesome experience would be the energizer to which I would return when I needed strength or encouragement. Today it is still the source of my drive and zest for life. I stay in touch with this dynamic inner power, which lies dormant within, just waiting to be called forth.

I find that I am also more tolerant and patient, more caring and loving, if I take the time to get in touch with my deeper self. I am then acting from the core of who I am, rather than from just below the surface. I find my quiet time alone with God downright essential for the development of my inner universe. Quiet time bestows the wisdom needed in my search for meaning. I find this gift of solitude one of the richest paths in providing peace in an otherwise hectic world.

I have discovered through the years that life in the Spirit is an adventure. God is a God of surprises and you never know what is just around the corner. Everything is shot through with divinity and so holds enormous potential and excitement. When I am open to this faith vision, I am able to live on a deeper level. I am overwhelmed to this day when I recount the many blessings I have been given. My praise knows no bounds.

# Expectation

*Thanks for what has been, Yes to the future.*
—DAG HAMMARSKJÖLD

A refreshing and liberating freedom, complemented with responsibility, was an outcome of this experience. I now realize that a relationship with God is far more than the keeping of rules and regulations. The latter start us on our way but they cannot possibly capture the love response of a true relationship.

This awareness of God's presence in my life, this assurance that I am loved unconditionally, has enabled me to be more open to encountering God in a multitude of ways. These ways would have been closed to me before, so narrow was my vision. Today I see God's presence in great abundance—in my caring husband, a trustworthy friend, a compassionate listener, a thought-provoking book, the impish smile of a grandchild, the green of a golf course, the glittering trees after a winter ice storm, a strength that springs forth in time of crisis. There is no aspect of creation that is void of the presence of God. It is only limited by my perceptions.

I know experientially that God loves me in spite of my sinfulness. I wait in expectation for the love to be further revealed in my life, and I am always pleasantly surprised. By sharing my story, I am trying to acknowledge the tremendous gift I have been given through no merit of my own. My faith has been deepened beyond my wildest expectations and my hope knows no bounds. I truly pray that the sharing of my gift will inspire others to let God touch their lives.

When encountering the incomprehensible mystery, the following quote captures beautifully the trust that is needed: "When we come to the edge of our light, we will either step over onto something solid or we will be taught how to fly." I pray that my story will encourage you to trust. The incomprehensible mystery invites. Accept the invitation to journey with God. Step into the unknown. You will not be disappointed.

## Response to Story Two

• "Be still and know that I am God." Do you truly believe these words? What interferes with your efforts to set up a prayer time for yourself? What can you do about it?

• What in your life reveals to you that you are loved by God? How have you responded to this grace? What do you do to raise your awareness of God's presence in your life?

• "The prayers of the righteous person are powerful." What is your reaction when your prayers are not answered according to your plan? When prayer is dry and you feel abandoned by God, what do you do? How faithful are you to prayer when this happens? What motivates your prayer life: consolations in prayer, fidelity to prayer, need, fear, gratitude, duty?

• If someone were to ask you why you trust God, how would you answer?

• "You may be the only 'Bible' some people will ever read." How does your life reveal God's unconditional love for people?

• In your life how have you experienced the hidden God? The humor of God? The Enabling God? The God of Unconditional Love? The Mysterious God?

•Which of the following best describes your prayer and why? moving God to action, you to action; fishing, golfing, or any other secular activity; a hunger or yearning of the human spirit; a gift freely given; exciting or adventuresome; dry, arid, difficult; stillness or presence; imagining yourself in a gospel story; writing or keeping a journal; mystery.

## Let Us Pray...

*This is what the Lord asks of you, only this: to act justly, love tenderly, and walk humbly with your God.* —MICAH 6:8

My Lord and God, thank you for loving me even when I ignore you. Open my ears so that I might clearly hear the call to prayer. You are forever inviting, but I am forever neglecting to respond. I have many good excuses: I am so busy running the kids, I have social obligations that must be met, I'm active in the community. I'm sure you have heard them all before.

I have good intentions, but by evening I'm so tired. Renew my Spirit so that I may take a deeper interest in my prayer life. Help me to put it higher on my priority list. Allow me to see how much it benefits me to spend time with you. I trust you will answer this prayer knowing it will make me more aware of your presence in my life. Amen.

Story Three

# Wrestling with Cancer

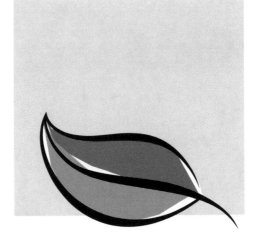

# The Battle Begins

*God does not want us to be burdened because of sor-*
*rows and tempests that happen in our lives because*
*it has always been so before miracles happen.*
                                    —JULIAN OF NORWICH

In the fall of 1975 with the encouragement of my husband, Bob, I had enrolled in college to get my Bachelor's degree. I found the classes stimulating and thought-provoking. Indeed, college for me was addictive. In 1983 I was still in school, though the classes I took now were part of my Doctoral program. I could only attend part-time since we were also raising our family. I had discovered that the two careers complemented each other. My broader vision gave me a better understanding for raising children, while family life kept me rooted in reality. I had the best of both worlds.

My battle with cancer began that year, 1983. I had a lump on my head that was diagnosed as a cyst. My understanding was that this would not be a problem unless the lump started to hurt or change shape. These symptoms did eventually appear, but since I was in the middle of a school semester, I decided to wait until the end of the term to have the lump removed. Cancer never entered my mind.

There are three comments I remember distinctly from that first encounter with cancer. My doctor had sent me to a surgeon to have the cyst removed. I was under local anesthetic, and so I heard the sur-

45

geon repeatedly say, "This does not look good. This really does not look good." Maybe he thought I was in "la-la" land and could not hear him. However, I remember this comment clearly, for I marked it as the beginning of my ongoing battle with cancer.

The surgeon, upon completion of the procedure, did not refer to his comment at all. He was a surgeon. It wasn't his place, I suppose, to diagnose a cancerous condition. He did insist, though, that I see my family doctor that same day. Naturally I knew that something was wrong. However, I chose to discuss it with the doctor with whom I felt most comfortable.

The surgeon had evidently called ahead, for I had no trouble getting in to see my doctor that same afternoon. He referred to the telephone call from the surgeon and so I asked him to tell me the truth. This was my life and I wanted to be informed. The only urgency in my voice was the need to know. His reply was blunt, "You have a blood disease." I remember that even that information did not upset me. I looked upon it simply as a medical condition that would require treatment.

The third comment I clearly remember was later that same Friday afternoon. I had a scheduled session with my spiritual director, Fr. Tony, and so I told him the news, but still with no deep concern. When I mentioned to him that perhaps this disease, this cancer, would be localized, he gently replied, "Bev, blood isn't localized." His comment did not shake me either, for I had still not comprehended the seriousness of the situation. My optimistic nature had just taken over. It had been a very busy and full day, and I had not had time yet to reflect deeply on these matters.

My husband Bob had a fishing trip planned for the weekend. I, too, had plans. I would spend the weekend with a friend, MaryAnne, while Bob was gone. I decided not to tell him before he left. There was no reason to worry him over nothing. We would have plenty of time to discuss what action we would take when he came home on Sunday. He left for his weekend excursion content that all was well.

That Friday evening my friend had a meeting, and I looked forward to the peace and quiet after such a hectic day. As I grew quiet and centered down, the impact of the day's events finally hit me full force. I had the dreaded big "C," the word that carried such gloom and doom. I had cancer!

I panicked. Would I survive? I still had children at home. Would I live long enough to raise them? How would they get along without a mother? I also thought about Bob. My death would be unfair to him. He was too young to be widowed. I had never dealt with cancer before and I had no idea what to expect. It was an unknown to me and I was petrified.

By the time MaryAnne came home, I was a basket case. Even though it was eleven at night, she called my spiritual director and we went over to see him. The three of us talked a long time and I began to regain my balance. As we prayed together, my fears dissipated and my spirits bounced back. I left with the thought that God is with me and together there is nothing we can't handle. I had, with the help of friends, once more regained my composure.

I cannot stress enough the importance of a support community. God is so amazingly present in the people who are part of my life. I draw my strength from them. I truly believe this community of family and friends is an invaluable gift given to me by God. It is due to their prayers and support that I am able to deal with cancer as easily as I do. The medicine heals the body, but it is the support community who keeps the spirit alive and well.

Later that month, Fr. Tony and MaryAnne planned a prayer service. A group of church friends came together to ask for God's healing. Each laid their hands on me and said a prayer over me. I was then anointed with oil in the form of a cross on my forehead. I was deeply touched by the love and concern shown me. Once the Spirit is rolling, there is no limit to what can be accomplished, and the Spirit was truly present at that service. I believe a miracle took place that evening, for the cancer was found only on the lump on my head. It was diagnosed as Non-Hodgkins Lymphoma. It was not as deadly as other forms of cancer. True, there was no cure, but it could be treated with chemotherapy and put in remission. My prayers were answered. I would live to see my last two children reach adulthood.

One of the most surprising aspects with this first encounter with cancer was the loss of hair. I never dreamed this would be so traumatic. I thought I had reconciled myself to the fact that I would have to wear a wig. After all, I had all this theological training and was not deeply immersed in the material world, or so I thought. I was confident that this side effect would pose no problem for me. But when my hair started falling out as I showered, just from the pressure of the water, it was startling. It demanded my attention. It dramatically drove home how little control I had in this situation. I dealt with this issue, but much to my astonishment, with difficulty.

Cancer would accompany me through my life, but it would turn out to be a companion that revealed the outrageous love of my God for me. To realize that cancer could be a source of grace, however, was a lesson learned with great difficulty. In the years to come my demands on God would be great, but nonetheless graciously fulfilled.

# The Healing Process

In 1989 cancer was diagnosed again. This time it appeared around my eye. The doctor operated to remove the lump and this was followed with radiation. This lump was so close to the eye that it was necessary to pinpoint exactly where to radiate. To do this a mask was formed to fit my face. When I went for treatment, this mask, which was then placed over my face, was bolted to the table. In this way I could not, even inadvertently, move my head during the radiation treatment. The eye was safely guarded.

Because I am also a diabetic, I would later lose fifty percent of the sight in this left eye. The combination of diabetes and radiation is not a good mix. However, at the time of the radiation treatment the diabetes connection was still an open question. I later learned, as part of a test study at the University of Michigan Hospital involving the interaction of diabetes and radiation, that some diabetics were not affected in this way. Once again life challenged me with its mysterious ways. I would search to find meaning in all of this—but it would take time and require patience.

It was during this eye treatment that I further developed my "inner universe." I have a tendency to be claustrophobic so I would mentally remove myself during the time my masked face was bolted to the table. Since I am an avid golfer, one of the places I chose to go was the golf course. I would practice my swing and play the golf holes over in my mind. This mental activity truly did improve my actual golf game. Needless to say, in this mind game I always turned in a good score!

Another place to which I would mentally escape was my sacred space. This God-space within, this inner universe, can take whatever shape we give it. My God-space took the form of a valley. This technique is simply an image aid in helping us interact with a sometimes mysterious and unseen God. I need only be still and enter my valley to encounter my God who is forever present there waiting for me. It is a comforting and healing place of retreat.

Science today is finally recognizing the interconnectedness of body and mind. Dr. Bernie Siegel writes in *Love, Medicine, and Miracles,* "Visualization takes advantage of what might also be called a weakness of the body: it cannot distinguish between a vivid mental picture and an actual physical experience." I had once again stumbled onto something which was later affirmed through reading. I had been visiting my valley on a regular basis for some time, not realizing how beneficial it was to me, not only spiritually but also physically.

I need to describe my valley in order to explain how I use the healing process of the mind with the healing process of chemotherapy. I slowly descend to the center of myself, my inner universe. As I pass through darkness when descending, I repeat the name of Jesus over and over. This helps me clear my mind of everyday distractions. The darkness then gives way to white fluffy clouds. When passing through the clouds I attempt once again to leave behind any problems or questions that are present. My goal at this point is to simply enter the valley in a peaceful state of mind.

The clouds begin to dissipate and a sunny, lush green valley appears before me. It is surrounded by mountain ranges, which assure its solitude. The fields are filled with a mixture of flowers, all kinds of animals, and a variety of trees. Peacefulness permeates everything.

The path that winds through the valley leads to a mountain stream to which I have assigned great healing powers. As I walk to the stream

I am greeted by my support community, living and dead. My parents, family, and friends bless me as I pass between them to reach the healing waters.

I enter the water where Jesus is waiting for me. As I feel the water pass over and around me, I visualize the dreaded cancer cells flowing out of my body carried away by the current of the stream. I stay with this picture as long as possible, allowing the water to repeatedly cleanse my body. There is a "laying on of hands" by Jesus to assure me that the disease is leaving my body. When we emerge from the stream, I see myself dressed in a white robe, which represents wholeness to me. I feel refreshed in mind and body.

Jesus and I then continue down the path. As we do so, family and friends are left behind, for this is the place of my inner solitude. They are present only at the mountain stream during the healing process. In the far distance a giant oak tree stands and that is our destination. It is there on a swing that Jesus and I continue our conversation in private.

I have learned to use this healing technique, not only while receiving chemotherapy, but whenever I feel that my body or spirit is in need. This visit to my inner universe never fails to renew my strength. I am always left with a pervasive peace and confidence that healing was—and is—taking place, whether it be physical or spiritual.

Before this second bout with cancer, friends and family never entered my valley. However, I find that with each new circumstance in my life my valley takes on new form and, as such, never becomes a stagnant place. Rather, it is a vibrant and growing prayer valley with a dynamic all its own.

I want to stress at this point that prayer can take many forms. I am simply describing here a way of praying with images that works for me. In other situations, just sitting in the presence of God is what may be needed. And yet again, formal prayer may be what some people need. The invitation is to pray—in the way that is best for you.

The German theologian Karl Rahner comments on the need of the modern person. He writes: "When we say that prayer is necessary, we mean necessary for the highest part of man's nature, and just as the highest part of man—his soul—is often ignored, so too is prayer." One of my favorite authors, Abraham Heschel, states it more poetically: "All things have a home: the bird has a nest, the fox has a hole, the bee has a hive.

A soul without prayer is a soul without a home" (*Wisdom of Heschel*).

God is constantly trying to communicate with us, trying to touch us and be present to us. All that is required on our part is to sit in stillness and listen. True, in a noisy world this can be difficult. However, to give our soul a "home," we must accept the challenge.

# New Perspectives

*It is so difficult to believe because it is so difficult to suffer.* —PASCAL

Even though I had in the past recognized that God's love was always present, I needed at this time to open that question once again. How we humans need affirmation! God is so patient with us. Each time, though, that I struggle through my doubts and questions, a new perspective always surfaces. God reveals more to me probably because my ability to understand is deepening. My question at that time was, in light of my situation, how did love and power combine to produce cancer and chemotherapy?

I related this question of God's power to the issue of love. After much prayer and study, I was finally led to understand that God's "power" stops at the beginning of our freedom. Does that sound blasphemous? Yet it is the way that God created the world. God has such tremendous respect for the freedom and dignity of the human person that we are not forced to return the love. God invites us to love and leaves us free to respond! It is the intrinsic nature of love to give freely of itself. It can't be authentic love if it is imposed, even if the "imposer" is the transcendent God. That is why the greatest gift we have to offer is ourselves—freely given.

Again I turn to Abraham Heschel who captures so beautifully the dignity of the human person: "Reverence for God is shown in our reverence for man. The fear you must feel of offending or hurting a human being must be as ultimate as your fear of God. An act of violence is an act of desecration. To be arrogant toward man is to be blasphemous toward God" (*Wisdom of Heschel*). With such a lofty view of who the human person is, freedom to respond to God must be part of our very nature.

The resolution of this love and power question gave me peace. The God of love had patiently given me a new and deeper perspective on our relationship. I now viewed the God of power as the enabling force in transforming this situation. This truly would be a powerful movement. This could be accomplished by the choice of my attitude in dealing with cancer. I could choose to be angry with God, blame God for what I was going through. I could refuse to make a loving response to my situation. God would not force the correct and proper response from me. I was free to wallow in the downside of this burden.

On the other hand, I could respond with trust to the God who loved me and had demonstrated this repeatedly in my life. I could opt to stress the good that can be found in any situation if we are open to look for it. I could choose to emphasize the positive. After all, the bouts of cancer did make me reflect on the ultimate meaning in life. They did lead me to new insights which broadened my image of God. It gave me a deeper appreciation of family and friends. It forced me to live in the present moment. I did not waste time regretting the past or waiting impatiently for the future. I lived every moment of my life fully, whether it was on the golf course with friends, celebrating birthdays with family, or knee-deep in chemotherapy. Furthermore, if I did not give cancer the power, it could not alter the deepest part of who I am. It could not negatively affect my relationship with my God. And if my relationship with God was healthy, so were all other relationships.

I also believe that my cancer has affected my family in a positive way, because I now take none of them for granted. I recognize that life is fragile and precious. The shadow of death on the horizon truly raises awareness of how to live life authentically. It sounds trite, but I would not be the person I am today without my "burden" of cancer.

To live is to interact with the mystery that is our God. I believed God could cure this cancer rather than send it into remission. It was just that God mysteriously remained silent on the matter in my case. God chose to heal and love me in a different way. I chose to accept this reality, confident that I was loved. I would trust my God, knowing that I could not see the total picture. I chose to believe that God's way was more effective in helping me reach my ultimate goal of life. I put my hope in Jesus and chose to use the cancer as a way to enhance our relationship.

As I was attempting to integrate these ideas into my life, God once again gave me affirmation that I was on the right track. My thoughts went back to an experience I had had with my youngest son. At the time Aaron was about five years old and he had done something wrong for which I had just corrected him. He was stomping out of the kitchen when he said, "I don't love you anymore." I was not about to stoop to his level, so I blew him a kiss. He ducked saying, "It missed." I saw the smile on his face as he continued on his way. I couldn't help but laugh as I thought about his quick reaction. I recognized, though, how that episode captured so well our relationship with God. God is forever throwing us kisses and we are the ones ducking. We are the ones putting up the obstacles to God's unconditional love. Our attitude alone can distort the vision God is attempting to give us.

Even though I question and doubt continuously, or so it seems, God is ever there to help me through my struggle. An unconditional love is a wonderful love for people who repeatedly fall and stumble. This type of love is absolutely necessary. We are finite and are in the process of becoming all that we can be. God's love affirms us each step of the way. This unconditional love is the fuel that feeds this "becoming" process, even when that process takes us through a minefield of questions and doubts.

# The Dividing Line

*Faith is being sure of what we hope for and certain of what we do not see.* —HEBREWS 11:1

Cancer appeared again in 1991. This lump was found in the neck area. As I had chosen to use my struggle with cancer as a way to God, peacefulness settled over me. I still heartily believe God does not send sickness, but can use it to bring us closer to our potential. God's love for us is so great that any and every situation can be used to raise our awareness of it. Again it bears repeating that God can bring good out of any evil or sickness. This is such a tremendous message of hope that it needs to be shouted from the housetops.

Cancer struck again in 1993 and 1994. I would, once again, have to deal with the chemotherapy treatment which brought about the upset stomach, the loss of hair necessitating the need for a wig, the fatigue that accompanied the cure, the time-consuming trips to the doctor's office. By the time these two episodes passed, my body was very weak. I was experiencing my humanity deeply.

I have kept a journal for the last twenty-five years. It was in reading over my journal that I recognized a gradual awareness unfolding. I had always considered that first bout of cancer a fluke. I would take the chemotherapy, clear up this mistake, and get on with my life. I retained this mindset even with the second and third occurrences. I had not yet crossed what I call "the invisible dividing line of life." I was still indestructible. So strong was my positive life force that I felt nothing could hold me down indefinitely. I would always be able to get the best of any situation. And so with every episode of cancer my optimism would surface and I would truly believe we had sent it into remission forever.

However, I noticed in reading my journal that this time my outlook was slowly changing, taking on a new perspective. This was the fifth time I would deal with cancer, and though I am an optimist, I am also a realist. I recognized that I would not live forever. I was indeed mortal. I was a finite being. I had stepped over the dividing line. The thought of death entered the picture for the first time. I want to stress, though, that I was not morbid about this. These reflections did not put a damper on my life. Rather, it was almost a peaceful coming-to-terms with reality. It was more an acknowledgment that death is part of the life process. With this mindset, life simply was to be appreciated and celebrated to the fullest.

It is strange, though, the directions the mind takes when it finally acknowledges its mortality. I explored the ultimate question: is there life after death? For the first time there were no burning questions, absolutely no doubt. I knew with certainty there was a core "I" that would survive physical death. The unconditional love of our God demanded my continuance. I was surprised at how quickly this issue had been resolved. I was totally at peace with my world.

The more I pursued the issue, the more exciting it became. Death could be a downright adventure. I would finally get a chance to ask my questions. What happened with the Holocaust? Why such suffering? How can people be so inhumanly cruel? Can the divinity in people be crushed to extinction? The questions then took a different turn. Is there life on other planets? Will contact be made in the future? Will the universe go on forever? As I continued down this path, my thoughts turned to family. Would I be able to make contact with them after death? Would I be able to protect them from harm? God and I would have a great deal to talk about in the hereafter!

I dealt with the ultimate questions, but the finite side of me also demanded attention. I was slowly learning that I was not pure spirit,

I was also very human. When I stepped over that dividing line and death entered the picture, I became concerned about what I was leaving behind spiritually, but also materially. Which pieces of my jewelry would I leave to my daughter and daughters-in-law? What could I leave my sons and son-in-law for a keepsake? I searched for something meaningful to give to each grandchild. Again, this was not a morbid activity. It was just something I wanted to do, and I enjoyed assigning the sentimental pieces I would leave behind.

Bob and I also felt certain steps should be taken. We set up a living trust. A Durable Power of Attorney was made out by both of us. Neither of us wanted to be kept alive with machines. Death was not imminent, but I felt comfortable dealing with these issues at this time. There was no deep sadness connected to this. It was just a duty that had to be done. I was simply putting my affairs in order.

Don't get me wrong; I do still wrestle with my disease. I have my down days, and I must deal with depression. It is simply part of the human condition. Sickness can wear you down, and after sixteen years it has taken its toll on me. I simply refuse to let it get the upper hand. I give depression its due, let it reign for a day, and then I dethrone it. It deserves no more of my time.

Depending on the grip of the darkness, however, there are times when it is more difficult to shed the mood than at other times. The secret is to address the downward spiraling immediately. Do not allow it to send down roots and thus lodge itself firmer in your psyche. For me, people are the vehicle I need to break the grip of a down day. I will meet a friend for coffee or for lunch. Sometimes just making contact by phone will snap me out of it. I have never failed, though, to rise up out of a dark mood when I am able to mingle with the "sparks of divinity."

Although it appears that cancer has dominated my life for the last sixteen years, this is not totally accurate. I have refused to give it that much power. The main focus has been the healthy times, not the sick ones. It is true that the cancer episodes bring the ultimate questions to the forefront, for it is then that I am forced to acknowledge my mortality.

In truth, however, cancer has been squeezed between normal family events. Through my six bouts, children have graduated and gone to college. Marriages have taken place and grandchildren have been born and baptized. Parents have died and so have friends who battled cancer and lost. Birthdays have been celebrated and losses mourned. Vacations have been taken and golf tournaments played. New friendships have been formed while old ones deepened. The family home was sold and a new one built in the country. Life has moved along smoothly in spite of my disease.

As I describe this aspect of my journey, it sounds so easy, but this is not necessarily the case. Recognizing my task in life—meaningfully interweaving the cancer with the joyous events taking place—was a gradual unfolding process. Upon first encounter, life's lessons are rarely grasped in their entirety. To this day I continue to discover how I can better integrate cancer into my life. Without fail, though, God gives me the vision and courage to accomplish this.

When I read my journals, I recognize that faith is the stance required of me. Faith helps me to recognize the light. Yes, there are times when my faith becomes so tarnished with doubt and darkness that it is difficult for the light to shine through. At these times, prayer and solitude are essential to keep it shining. If wisdom is to accompany me on my journey, the brightness of God's love must be the dominant light in my life.

Faith represents the ability to stand on the edge of the abyss and fall into the unknown, confident that God will be there to catch me. Faith is surrendering to the mystery that is life, believing that an unconditional love is the underpinning of that life. Faith is saying yes to the dying process, knowing that God not only accompanies me, but also participates in every movement of my life. Yes, faith is the stance I needed, and I would work diligently to deepen it.

# The Uphill Struggle

There are no easy ways, there are no simple solutions. What comes easy is not worth a straw. It is a tragic error to assume that the world is flat, that our direction is horizontal. The way is always vertical. It is either up or down; we either climb or fall. Religious existence means struggle uphill.

—ABRAHAM HESCHEL

In 1995 cancer again surfaced. This time the enlarged nodes were found in my chest and abdomen. The c-scan also showed an enlarged spleen. True, the same old questions and doubts surfaced, but with each passing cancer episode, they have slowly lost their power and impact. This time they were quickly swept away. However, as this episode unfolded, the grumbling would return. God's patience is eternal.

I had asked God for a reprieve from cancer. I needed a break. I had dealt with this disease off and on for sixteen years. I thought God and I had struck a deal. So when it resurfaced again so soon, I felt betrayed. God had not kept to the bargain. I guess when we are tired and not feeling very well, it is human nature to try to bargain with God. The old outdated memory tapes were playing in my head. I had bargained with God many times in the past. Ideas once held die hard.

Not only was I disappointed because cancer popped up so soon again, but my first round of chemotherapy was accompanied by a sore throat which made it that much worse. The second cycle of chemotherapy was immediately followed by a burning, itching rash.

I began to feel sorry for myself. I did not need these extra burdens. Wasn't it enough that I had cancer and was going through the chemotherapy for the sixth time? Did I have to have these other annoying symptoms?

I prayed for a miracle. None came. Both annoyances ran their course. Did God hear my prayer? I truly believe this was the case, but I was just in a griping mood. I know some people are delivered from their sickness while others are not. Whenever I experience these times of unanswered physical deliverance, I turn to my journal and allow my memory banks to take over. I recall the many times God has revealed unconditional love for me in a thousand different ways. I am always overwhelmed with shame when in the midst of my grumbling I remember God's tender care for me throughout my life. I have learned, and continue to learn, that accepting and surrendering to the mystery in life is a big part of the human task.

The cancer treatment continued, but halfway through there was trouble with my veins. I took chemotherapy five days in a row and then was off for three weeks. Needless to say I had to be inserted with needles these five days. It was determined a port would be beneficial so I underwent minor surgery. This allowed easy access for the intravenous chemotherapy drip. With the port in place, the rest of the treatment went along smoothly.

When taking chemotherapy, there is a nadir period when the patient has no resistance to germs. They are advised to stay home to avoid catching something that would hinder treatment and the healing process. A couple of months during this time, my husband had a cough from congestion in his chest, two sons had the flu, and the youngest grandchildren had colds. I humorously wondered if God was tired of my grumbling, for I had been exposed to all these things and never caught any of them. I quietly returned thanks for the protection I had been given once again.

With my first five bouts of cancer, the routine had always been the same. Cancer raises its ugly head. The c-scan reveals where it is hiding this time. The decision is made as to what kind of chemicals to give, what strength the drugs should be, and how often chemotherapy should be given. The program is then set in motion. Once the chemotherapy is completed, the cancer again goes into remission.

This time would be no different, I thought. I had learned a great deal since my first encounter with cancer about the chemotherapy treatment, and also about myself.

I was sure that with the medical field offering me chemotherapy; my visualization with the healing waters of my inner universe; the prayers of my support community; and the openness born out of my optimistic nature, the c-scan after my six-cycle treatment would show me once more to be free and clear of cancer. I was looking forward to a remission time when I could put hospital and doctors behind me for awhile.

Can you imagine my disappointment when the word came back that the tumors were still there. I was very down. This was supposed to be the rest and relaxation period. But once again a book touched my life. I had just finished reading Richard Rohr's *Job and the Mystery of Suffering.* In my notes I found this statement, "You cannot solve the problem, you can only live the mystery." It resonated deep within. The co-partnership concept came to mind, and so I chose to keep an optimistic attitude and open myself to what lay ahead.

It was determined that I would need to take more chemotherapy. We would evaluate after each treatment and decide on a course of action. I knew that meant more c-scans, more blood tests, more hospital visits. However, I had said "yes" to the future, and so I was ready to see where this episode would lead. It turned out to be quite an adventure.

This time the cancer had taken a different unknown course. I would have to be creative in my response. I turned to my quiet time to put balance in my life. This time alone allowed me to stand back and reflect on my life and the course it was now taking. I recalled Viktor Frankl's concept that if you have a "why" you can endure almost any "how." I had plenty of "why" in my life (*Man's Search for Meaning*).

I decided I would enjoy the present moment to the fullest. My husband and family took center stage. I observed with amusement and pride my own children parenting their children. I loved watching the "becoming process" of my grandchildren. I noticed with joy how each one was developing his or her own unique personality.

I relished the stimulating thoughts produced by a good book. Even the flowers and greenery of summer became more vivid. The time spent golfing with family and friends was energy-giving. Searching for truth and meaning took on deeper significance. Each moment held something special as I recognized my limitedness. Yes, I had plenty of "why." I would survive the "how" the future held.

After another cycle of chemotherapy, there was still no improvement. In 1996 I was sent to the University of Michigan Cancer Center. There, after much consultation on their part—and prayer on mine—it was determined that I would be a good candidate for an experimental program called Radiotherapy.

In order to quality, I had to meet certain criteria. A bone marrow test was needed. The tainted cells in the bone marrow had to be less than twenty-five percent. I passed the test, but the procedure left me hurting. My hip ached every time I took a step and since it was summer that meant golf and a lot of steps. This was an unusual by-product of the test. I was told it was nothing serious and would pass. It did, but it took about three months.

Another complication arose when my red cell blood count started to dip. I had very little energy. I was put on Prednisone to help raise it, but it would take quite awhile. I had dropped below eight, half of what the doctors wanted it to be. As the summer of 1996 unfolded, I began to find it tiring to even walk across the room. I rested and slept as much as possible, but I would not give up my golf. It helped to keep life in perspective, to keep balance in the midst of a great deal of chaos.

Paul Pearsall in his book *Making Miracles* has a unique perspective on the difficult times, those periods of sickness and darkness that arise in one's life. He writes, "Chaos shuffles the cards for us so that we don't have to cope with the trauma of choosing the nature or the timing of our crises. We don't and can't tell the universe what to do, we can only be a part of the doing." It is enough for me to handle being "a part of the doing." To select the what and when of a crisis would be an unbearable choice.

Thomas Merton explains exactly what my "doing" entails: "The Christian must not only accept suffering, he must make it holy. Nothing so easily becomes unholy as suffering."

By "holy" I took him to mean that somehow we must bring good out of it. We must allow God to transform suffering into a meaningful experience. To do this, openness is required on our part; an openness that will let in a broadened interpretation of life; an openness that is permeated with prayer.

Merton warns us that it is not an easy task but it is a challenge that we must accept if we want to live our life in light rather than darkness, in meaningfulness rather than absurdity.

# The God of Surprises

*Be prepared at all times for the gifts of God and be ready always for new ones. For God is a thousand times more ready to give than we are to receive.*

—MEISTER ECKHART

I am a member of a four-woman scramble golf team and in 1996 we won the county tournament which entitled us to go to the State Finals at Boyne Mountain. However, we had won the county tournament in the spring when I was feeling better. The State Tournament was held in the fall. Now I was hurting. I was not strong and I had zero endurance. I couldn't possibly go to Boyne in this condition. I couldn't even play nine holes of golf, let alone eighteen for two continuous days.

I wrote in my journal at this time, "I am angry. After all I have been through I am not going to be able to enjoy the one weekend I had so been looking forward to all summer. I don't understand. I am terribly disappointed. I feel abandoned. However, I will offer praise anyway, Lord, not because I feel like it but because it is what I am supposed to do." I was trying to be faithful to my Christic vision but it was not easy. Out of a sense of duty I offered a prayer of praise, but the intense disappointment was ever-looming. However, the God of surprises had something wonderful in store for me. I believe that because I tried to remain open, tried to live up to my part of this partnership, struggled to actuate the possibilities in my life, I contributed to the surprising gift I was about to be given.

With me on the team were Melany Tingley, Bernell Wood, and Christine Topley. They were wonderful. In spite of the fact that we would not be competitive, they refused to go without me. They insisted we go together if only for the companionship. I could ride the cart. I could help on the par three holes. They certainly wouldn't need my drive. My iron play would be my contribution. It didn't matter, we were going just for the fun of it. My disappointment faded as I prepared to go to Boyne with the team. I thought to myself that God had come through once again. I would have my weekend despite the cancer. I returned thanks for the gift of Boyne, but I didn't take into account the creativity of our God.

You must understand the weakening condition I was in to appreciate the extraordinary event that was about to take place. I was extremely tired. I did not tee off on every hole for I simply did not have the stamina. I decided I would save my energy and use it where I felt I might be able to contribute. My red cell blood count was so low that I even had a difficult time breathing. But the team looked after me, and we were together having a good time.

As I stood on the par three eleventh hole to tee off, my teammates were giving me advice: swing out to the hole, use more club, take it back on the inside. We weren't competitive, but our pride urged us on to turn in the best score we could. I made a good swing and saw the ball hit the green. I was satisfied. I contributed. I then walked back to the cart where I could sit down. As I was putting my club away I heard the team yelling. I had made a hole-in-one! I did not see it go in, but I was ecstatic, exhausted as I was.

Unless you are a golfer you can't really appreciate this story. I had golfed for twenty-five years and this was my first hole-in-one. Most people golf all their lives and never achieve this feat. It also was special that it had happened at a State Tournament. As it turned out, we did not have a camera with us, but one of the team had a cell phone. I called home as soon as we walked off the green. I wanted to share this wonderful time immediately. Bob had always been with me during the difficult cancer times. I wanted him to share in the excitement and joy of this moment. It was a day I would never forget. We celebrated the rest of the weekend.

A hole-in-one is so rare that they are always acknowledged at the golf banquet in the evening. Of the five hundred plus golfers, men and women, who were at Boyne Mountain that weekend, only one other person and I recorded a hole-in-one. We were applauded, but I was given a standing ovation when the audience was told of my struggle with cancer. The story was especially interesting because this tournament was sponsored by the American Cancer Society. Pictures were taken and the story was written up in their monthly newsletter. Our score would not win us the tournament, but that weekend was one of the best times we had ever had.

In the midst of such chaos it was comforting and consoling to experience such a gift. God had not only cared for me, but made the weekend exciting and joyful for my team who could not be competitive because of me. In my reflections, I took note of the fact that the Bible was not the only place that had a story with a rainbow at the end.

# Broadened Horizons

Once back home the struggle with cancer went on. Another bone marrow test was needed for me to gain entry into the radiotherapy program.
My cells had to emit a strong signal so that the therapy would work. I
passed the test and this procedure did not leave me in pain. I was, however, still extremely tired. The Prednisone was not bringing my blood
count up fast enough, so I was given a blood transfusion.

The doctors consulted and decided that I needed at least one shot of
chemotherapy to keep the cancer at bay. It was so strong that even with
just one treatment, I again was in need of a wig. By this time there was
no trauma at seeing my hair fall out. It was just a nuisance to find it on
coats, collars, and chairs. I had come a long way since the first time I had
lost my hair. It was comforting to know that I was learning from my companion, cancer.

After the last bone marrow test, I was now ready for admittance into
the radiotherapy program. However, much to my surprise, another
obstacle appeared on the horizon. I would have to have my spleen out. I
was told it was so full of cancer that it had to be removed before anything
else could be done. I told myself that I could handle one more hurdle. I

was still riding high from the weekend at Boyne Mountain.

In November of 1996, my family and friends gathered with me for a healing Mass. My support community came through once again. Fr. Tony anointed me with oil and prayed over me. I am always in awe of the life-enhancing power I experience when the group gathers and prays with me. Armed with the knowledge that I was in God's tender care, I prepared for surgery.

The operation was to be a simple procedure. They had a new way of removing the spleen. Some small incisions were all that was needed. They crushed the spleen and took it out that way. The huge incision down the abdomen was a thing of the past. Two to three weeks was the recovery time. After all I had been through, I told myself that I could do this standing on my head. I would have it out before Thanksgiving and be up and running by Christmas.

As usual, things did not quite turn out the way I had planned. The spleen was much larger than anticipated, and before I died on the table from loss of blood, they had to resort to the "huge incision" of the past. It took me months to recover, complicated by the fact that I am a diabetic.

It has been said that a crisis brings out the best in people. In my experience, however, to deal with difficulty properly requires hope, faith, courage, perseverance, and much prayer. In *The Road Less Traveled,* M. Scott Peck writes that "it is only because of problems that we grow mentally and spiritually." I was surely having my share. With my problems, according to Peck, I must be learning by leaps and bounds. How could I be so lucky!

One day I was down in spirits but for good reason. I had an ugly scar down my middle plus three little scars at no extra charge. There seemed to be sagging skin everywhere due to weight loss, which made me look like an eighty-year-old. My back and side hurt and I had mysterious little protrusions all over my body. On top of all this, I had unaccounted-for burns under my breasts and on my back which required a great deal of attention so they would heal along with my incisions. Even though my husband was most attentive, I still felt alone in my suffering.

At times like this, the "shadow side" with all its doubts and fears mounts a fearsome attack. I was left wondering where God was in all of this. Anthony Padovano echoing Pascal writes: "There are times when the God of all-caring makes it difficult to believe." However, at this stage in my life, I knew that God was with me; I just couldn't recognize the presence.

Lately, whenever I am down and feeling sorry for myself, the thought crosses my mind that perhaps I am missing something. I know that I am blessed, but at down times I lose sight of that fact. Paul Pearsall reminded me of what was needed when he wrote: "Making miracles requires learning how to use our crisis and times of falling apart as vehicles for movement toward an ever-evolving and developing human spirit" (*Making Miracles*). I needed to regain a Christic perspective on life. I needed to use these experiences to help me get back in touch with what I knew I should ultimately be about—the search for meaning.

I had to gather my thoughts, to step back and look at the whole scene. Once again my quiet time provided the space I needed. With reflection I could more clearly see the presence of God. I saw the recovery of a diabetic from a serious operation with no complications. I remembered bone marrow tests and blood transfusions all resulting in good news. I recognized the support of the prayer group and caring friends that were always checking on me. My loving family and devoted husband always helped to speed the healing process. I was truly blessed. Thomas Merton was right when he wrote, echoing Socrates, that the unreflected life is not worth living. I used memory to put balance back into my life. I was returned to a healthy mental attitude.

I gleaned a great deal from this experience. I dedicated myself once more to deepening my relationship with the "Ineffable One." I was determined to diligently seek out how God was being revealed every time I had to go through something difficult. I would search for the meaningfulness in every experience. I would not expect God to be present in any particular way, but rather be open to God's surprises. I had never been this sick or hurt this much before. However, when I was put in touch with the total picture, I came away with renewed faith in my God and a deeper appreciation of God's love for me.

# The Adventure Deepens

God did not say: "You will not be tempted. You will not labor hard. You will not be troubled." But God did say: "You will not be overcome."

—JULIAN OF NORWICH

Recovery took some time, but by January, 1997 I was well on my way to feeling good. Could I go on a cruise with the family in February? It had been planned for a year and I was looking forward to it. I would take some books along to read and would be watchful of my activities. I consulted my doctor and she agreed that I needed the rest and relaxation. It would do me good. It looked as though my ordeal was finally winding down. I was elated.

That same evening I had a dream. In my dream I felt a "power surge" emerge from the depths. I don't exactly know how to explain the term "power surge." It is like a source of energy within me that suddenly the body is aware of. At times the energy makes itself felt by emitting powerful waves which rise up and then recede. It is not the everyday energy that people have but rather an explosive type of energy. Hence, I use the expression, "power surge."

The "power surge" produced an image of circular bouquets of flowers. They were shaped like a daisy with white centers and purple petals that were tinged with yellow at the tips. They were surrounded with a carpet of green grass. The colors were extremely vibrant. Perhaps that was due to the brilliant white light that permeated the whole scene. The picture then changed and tall stalks of flowers appeared, again with purple and yellow colors. The intense light was the constant in the two scenes. It was tremendously bright. An over-all feeling of joy and happiness was present throughout the dream. Then slowly the scene faded. Upon awaking, I still felt the serenity and peace the dream evoked.

I have always made a point to record any powerful experience. Dream or not, this was no exception. I wanted to capture what had really transpired. I wanted to grasp the core of the experience. After describing the incidentals, I wrote in my journal: "I sensed the powerful presence of God. A tremendous feeling of well-being in body and spirit settled over me."

This fascinating dream stirred my curiosity. I turned to John Sanford, a Jungian analyst who has written a great deal about dreams. He talks of an intelligence within the psyche which he does not hesitate to call God. He writes, "God is the name we give to the purposeful, numinous power that crosses our lives, and our dreams are one of the manifestations of this power" (*Dreams: God's Forgotten Language*). Confirmed in my interpretation, I chose to accept this dream as a gift from this "numinous power."

Maybe my body needed an energy boost. Maybe my psyche was recharging itself. After all I had been through, I didn't question, I simply basked in the feeling of well-being it produced. It renewed my attitude of surrender to the mystery that is life. And I would need this attitude to face the days ahead.

As the weeks passed, the excitement mounted as the day for the cruise approached. With high hopes we set sail. I was ready for this much-needed rest and relaxation. However, the second day into the cruise I realized something was going on with my body. I had developed some small red pimples which increased in number as the day went on. I needed once again to consult with a medical person. The ship's doctor wasn't sure what it was. I was a diabetic, had cancer, and had just been through an operation to have my spleen out. He was baffled. I was told to rest while he looked into it. It had been three weeks since our granddaughter had the chicken pox. Both the doctor and I did not think it was possible after that long a time to get them. Then Chad, our son, also broke out with these little red pimples. That settled it. You *can* get the chicken pox three weeks later!

The doctor told us the Caribbean culture had not been exposed to chicken pox. The ship's crew, therefore, were in danger. There were many ramifications that could occur from our condition. They attempted to put us off the ship on a small island but it had no hospital. Neither could they find any flight arrangements off the island. Chad and I, therefore, were quarantined in our cabins. Here I had put my trust in God for this cruise, and I ended up sicker than I was before I left. All I could think of was St. Teresa's humorous saying when she was in trouble: "If you (God) treat all your friends this way no wonder you have so few."

The humor in the situation soon faded. I was itchy and miserable. I know that God does not send sickness, but I was so disappointed and feeling so very sorry for myself that once again the outdated tapes started playing in my head. My positive attitude slipped away and the negative took over. Blame God! What kind of God did I serve? How was this showing me how much I am loved? Rapidly the downward spiraling began. How strong is the negative pull. God's patience is a needful grace!

I prayed for healing, but none came. I prayed for understanding, but no insights overwhelmed me. I searched for meaning, but could find nothing that made any sense. I picked up a book and read a quote from St. Teresa, "Consider the human weakness that is consoled by receiving help in time of need" (*Hidden Friends*). I could only think that I was receiving no such help.

Through the years I have come to realize that I must always keep a vigilant watch, for these dark moods have a way of sneaking up on me. When I am caught up in them, I cannot stress enough how blinding is the darkness that accompanies them.

I am amazed as I read my journal at how many times I have asked God to shower me with love and how many times my prayer was answered. Yet after only a few months, I ask God for the same thing again. After all I had been given, it shames me to acknowledge my lack of constancy and my shortsightedness. Poets say that gratitude is the memory of the heart. I must have had temporary amnesia! The only comfort I can take from this "amnesia" is that my continuous grumbling and complaining provide God with the opportunity to once more show outrageous love for me.

However, once more by way of books, God would provide the light I needed to find my way. Before the cruise I had just finished reading Richard Rohr's book, *Job and the Mystery of Suffering.* The only consolation his book gave me now was confirmation that God truly is a mystery. I began to reflect on that thought. I decided to work on my attitude. There is simply no human understanding of the eternal realm. The only way to relate to God is by loving. So I tried to accept my plight in a positive manner.

I did not understand the ways of the Lord, but I decided to thank God for this experience anyway. I really could not "own" such a prayer, but I had remembered that Karl Rahner once wrote that the only true prayer in any situation was one of praise. So I praised and thanked intellectually, knowing God would accept my intention. I was trying desperately to raise my awareness of God's presence in all this chaos. I was doing what the experts said to do. It might not have been coming from the heart but I was trying. Finally some sense of peace settled over me. However, the fullness of God's presence eluded me. I was still too deep in self pity.

If God wasn't going to lift this burden from me, I could at least expect to be consoled and commiserated with. I picked up another of the books I had brought on the cruise with me. It was *Stories of Awe and Abundance* by Jose Hobday. I read, "Be still and let God overwhelm you with love." I realized that I now had an opportunity for quiet and prayer, because the family group had gone ashore. An hour passed. Slowly I began to rise from the depths. I was finally beginning to see the light. Suddenly there was a knock at the door. When I answered it, from around the corner there appeared a hand holding a dish of chocolate covered strawberries. "Happy Valentines Day," a hesitant voice said. It was our cabin steward, too afraid to get close but wanting to lift my spirits. I felt the presence of God for which I had been so desperately searching.

All life is a matter of interpretation. One could chalk this up to coincidence. However I agree with Paul Pearsall in *Making Miracles* when he writes, "Be aware of the power of your observations of your life. Be alert for alternative or complementary explanations.... The higher the order or power of our coincidence, the more the universe is trying to draw attention to some aspect of your living, loving, and believing." Another may have chosen to label this episode coincidence, but I chose to interpret this event from the Christic point of view. This is how I find meaning in my life. It makes sense for me to believe that one of the ways God touches me is through ordinary experience, through ordinary people. When this occurs I credit God with acting anonymously. There simply have been too many times "coincidence" has touched into the core of who I am, and in so doing, renewed my effort to reach out for meaning in my life.

Since the Caribbean culture was very susceptible to the chicken pox, great care was taken to lessen their exposure to us. Most of the crew was of this culture, so our cabin steward had to be switched. Because I was quarantined to our cabin I had to use room service. I was itchy and still very miserable. I stayed in my robe for comfort and did not wear my wig. When I answered the door after ordering my dinner, I was surprised by the reaction of the waiter. He looked at me and his eyes grew as big as saucers. He took two steps back, extended the huge dinner tray, and simply said, "Take, take." He did not wait for his tip. He was halfway down the hall before I had even set the tray down. I was in my night clothes, completely bald, and covered with pox. I must have looked like death warmed over!

I can look back now and see the humor in the situation, but when you are mired knee-deep in pimples, baldness, and isolation, it is far more difficult. Through the years I have discovered that humor is a necessary requirement in dealing with life. It helps tremendously when reason does not suffice when encountering mystery.

Now the task before us was to get me home to my doctor. My husband was the rock through all of this. His constant assurance that I would be alright was comforting. In fact, I probably had the best possible scenario. I was quarantined to my room, but I did have family support, medical attention, room service, two large windows that gave me a view and sunlight, opportunity for plenty of rest which I needed, and time and quiet to read the thought-provoking books I had brought with me. By the time the cruise was over, my outbreak was under control. I not only survived this crisis but had further deepened my faith.

Through this experience I relearned two lessons: God is indeed mystery; and we do not have control of any situation; we can only control the attitude we choose to take. I vowed to be stronger next time and to be better at remembering that God is present in my times of difficulty as well as my times of joy.

We human beings are searchers after meaning, seekers all of our lives. We continually search, continually build on our development, continually work on our relationship with God for as long as we live. This adventure is endless, for our God is limitless mystery. If people are not searching for meaning in their experiences, they are missing the excitement, the challenge, and the treasure life can offer.

I wanted to learn, to deepen my relationship with God, but not on my vacation. I had it all wrong. When opportunity presents itself, you must take advantage of it or you stagnate. I almost look forward to the next difficulty to see what secrets or wisdom might be revealed, but I want to stress *almost*. Maybe I just don't trust myself to respond the way I know I should. I recognize that I am still very much in the becoming process.

# Trusting the Ineffable One

*When we regard God with awe and love God gently, our trust is never in vain. The more we trust and the more powerful this trust, the more we please and praise.*

—JULIAN OF NORWICH

My life experience has revealed to me that God is always there for me, walking every step of the way with me, giving me the courage and strength needed to address cancer each and every time it occurs. I have never had to carry the burden alone. I am in awe of a God who journeys with me in such an active way. It challenges me to live up to my side of this partnership.

We read in Isaiah 49:15, "Can a mother forget her infant, be without tenderness for the child of her womb; even should she forget, I will never forget you." In spite of my "memory lapses," my journals reveal that God's love has been bestowed on me over and over again through the years. This gift was graciously given to me even when I was not aware of the receiving. This is a tremendous insight into the kind of God we serve. It calls for me to be ever thankful and to praise always. Faith and trust grounded in this love makes cancer a companion rather than an enemy.

Quiet time is essential for creating my response to such powerful love. Prayer raises my consciousness and deepens my relationship with the "wholly other." Prayer produces the positive attitude and

Christic vision I need in times of difficulty. Time spent alone with the incomprehensible mystery is the underpinning of the inner peace that is present in my life.

I am always able to emerge from the chaos. I am always able to recognize the light despite the doubts, the fears, and the questions. This strongly demonstrates for me God's participation in my life. This positive attitude and inner peace astonishes even me. It is just as great a miracle to heal the mind as it is to heal the body. This is the miracle to which I bear witness!

At this time I am not a candidate for the radiotherapy program. I was informed in the spring of 1998 that I no longer met the time criteria required for this particular program. However, removing the spleen did wonders for me. My stamina returned and my golf game improved. My Spirit was renewed when I was able to make a trip to the Holy Land in the Fall of 1998. The pilgrimage was exceptionally meaningful and seemed a fitting conclusion to this particular chapter in my life.

Yes, the cancer remains, but we watch it closely. When it surfaces again we will deal with it again. I am in touch with an inner peace that assures me that I will be given the strength to do so.

In the meantime the trusting mode I find myself in allows me to adopt Thomas Merton's prayer in *Thoughts In Solitude* as my own:

My Lord God, I have no idea where I am going. I do not see the road ahead of me. I cannot know for certain where it will end. Nor do I really know myself, and the fact that I think I am following your will does not mean that I am actually doing so. But I believe that the desire to please you does in fact please you. And I hope I have that desire in all that I am doing. I hope that I will never do anything apart from that desire. And I know that if I do this you will lead me by the right road, though I may know nothing about it. Therefore I will trust you always though I may seem to be lost and in the shadow of death. I will not fear, for you are ever with me, and you will never leave me to face my perils alone.

•Identify some of the gifts and talents God has given you. How are you using them to reflect God to others?

•"God is constantly touching your life with caring presence." List ways that you have experienced this presence. Are you aware of God's presence even in the midst of difficulties? How might you become more aware?

•Can you recall a time when you encountered the God of surprises? Did it alter your view of how God acts in your life? Explain.

•Since death is part of the life process, what steps can you take to enhance your own peacefulness about it? Can you discuss death openly with your family and friends? If not, why?

•If you were to die tomorrow, what piece of advice would you give to those you love? Do you follow your own advice?

•When do you most experience God's presence or power in your life? Do you ever doubt God's participation in your life? What causes the doubts? What can you do to stop the "downward spiraling"? How can you turn this experience into an opportunity for growth?

•Using your imagination, picture a scene where Jesus and you are having a conversation. Share with him your difficulties, your concerns. What do you hear Jesus saying to you? What is your response? What do you say to Jesus? What do you think his response will be?

## Let Us Pray...

*Blessed is the person who perseveres under trials.*
—JAMES 1:12

O Lord, as I face the trials in my life, I pray that I might be pleasing to you in my attitude and actions. Help me to touch your presence within me, so that I may be in tune with the power that keeps the stars in place and the sun shining.

I know, Lord, that you walk with me during my difficulties, so raise my awareness of your presence. Sometimes I can be so blind. Give me the grace to recognize your caring love when I am knee-deep in my sufferings. Give me the inner peace and strength to face any outer turmoil. Confident this prayer will be answered, I thank you for this grace. Amen.

# Afterthoughts

I have chosen to share these three stories because of the depth of meaning they carry for me. They have shaped the vision I have of God, the world, and myself. I never again will be able to put parameters around my God and say this is where God fits. My God-image today is an open-ended one. This allows for the surprises God has in store for me.

The task I am called to is not great deeds, but great love. I have been given the power to avail myself of this dynamic love by simply being true to my humanity. God has placed within me a homing device, a yearning for the divine. If I follow it, I will reach my potential, my call to be one with the transcendent.

Because of these experiences, I stand in awe before the mystery that is our God. Even though I do not always understand God's workings, I can still trust because I know that I am loved.

I am also forced to acknowledge the tremendous dignity and authentic freedom accorded the human person when I recognize that the Ineffable One so readily interacts with me. From this I have also learned that sin is not an obstacle between God and us. When we focus on our sinfulness, ourselves, the spotlight is on the wrong image. God is the star of this drama.

My whole life has been intertwined with mystery, a mystery that has been subtle, hidden, humorous, full of surprises, yet always revealing a gentle caring presence. It is this insight that now sustains and directs my life.

I leave you to ponder the words of Abraham Heschel (from *Man Is Not Alone*), who expresses so beautifully the Ineffable in life:

Finite meaning is a thought we comprehend:
Infinite meaning is a thought that comprehends us;
Finite meaning we absorb;
Infinite meaning we encounter.
Finite meaning has clarity;
Infinite meaning has depth;
Finite meaning we comprehend with analytical reason;
To Infinite meaning we respond in awe.
Infinite meaning is uncomfortable,
Not compatible with our categories.
It is meaning wrapped in mystery.

# Suggested Readings

Campbell, Camille, Editor, *Meditations With Teresa of Avila,* Santa Fe, NM: Bear and Company, 1985.

Doyle, Brendan, Editor, *Meditations With Julian of Norwich,* Santa Fe, NM: Bear and Company, 1988.

Fox, Matthew, Editor, *Meditations With Meister Eckhart,* Santa Fe, NM: Bear and Company, 1988.

———————, *Original Blessing,* Santa Fe, NM: Bear and Company, 1983.

Frankl, Viktor, *Man's Search for Meaning,* Boston, MA: Beacon Press, 1959.

Fromm, Erich, *Man For Himself—An Inquiry Into the Psychology of Ethics,* New York, NY: Fawcett World Library, 1947.

Hammerskjöld, Dag, *Markings,* New York, NY: Alfred Knopf Company, 1966.

Heschel, Abraham Joshua (selected by Ruth Goodhill), *The Wisdom of Heschel,* New York, NY: Farrar, Straus & Giroux, 1970.

———————, *Man Is Not Alone—A Philosophy of Religion,* New York, NY: Farrar, Straus and Giroux, 1976.

———————, *Who Is Man,* Stanford, CA: Stanford University Press, 1963.

Hobday, Jose, *Stories of Awe and Abundance,* Kansas City, MO: Sheed and Ward, 1995.

James, William, *The Varieties of Religious Experience,* New York, NY: Collier Publishing (Division of Macmillan Publishing), 1961.

Jung, Carl, *Psychological Reflections,* Jolande Jacobi and R.F.C. Hull, Editors, Princeton, NJ: Princeton University Press, 1971.

Kelsey, Morton, *The Other Side of Silence,* New York, NY: Paulist Press, 1976.

Kierkegaard, Søren, *The Journals of Kierkegaard,* Alexander Dru, Trans., New York, NY: Harper and Bros., 1958.

Link, Mark, *Mission 2000—Praying Scripture in a Contemporary Way,* Allen, Texas: Tabor Publishing, 1992.

Lonergan, Bernard, *Method In Theology,* New York, NY: Seabury Press, 1972.

Merton, Thomas, *New Seeds of Contemplation,* New York, NY: New Directions, 1962.

_____, *No Man Is an Island,* Garden City, NY: Image Books, 1967.

_____, *Thoughts in Solitude,* New York, NY: Farrar, Straus & Giroux, 1956.

Otto, Rudolph, *The Idea of the Holy,* New York, NY: Oxford University Press, 1923.

Pearsall, Paul, *Making Miracles,* New York, NY: Prentice Hall Press, 1991.

Peck, Scott M., *The Road Less Traveled,* New York, NY: Simon and Schuster, 1978.

Progoff, Ira, *Jung, Synchronicity, and Human Destiny,* New York, NY: Dell Publishing, 1973.

Rahner, Karl, *On Prayer,* New York, NY: Paulist Press, 1958.

_____, *Words of Faith* (Alice Scherer, Editor), New York, NY: Crossroad Publishing Company, 1987.

Roberts, David, *Existentialism and Religious Belief,* New York, NY: Oxford University Press, 1957.

Rohr, Richard, *Job and the Question of Suffering,* New York, NY: Crossroad Publishing Company, 1997.

Sanford, John, *Dreams—God's Forgotten Language,* San Francisco, CA: Harper and Row, 1989.

Siegel, Bernie, *Love, Medicine and Miracles,* New York, hart NY: Harper and Row, 1986.

The Carmelites of Indianapolis, *Hidden Friends—Growing in Prayer,* Kansas City, MO: Sheed and Ward, 1995.

"Beverly Lancour Sinke has provided for us a wonderful gift of understanding the joy of an integrated life. With this compelling account of her journey she puts words to the indescribable path we all are called to walk. She helps us walk it in confidence and communion with our Sustainer."

Kevin W. Mannoia, President
National Association of Evangelicals


"This book is eminently readable, yet replete with the theological questions and background which affords the author the opportunity to put into words the anguish and wonder experienced by the heart and mind of every person faced with life-threatening illness. We journey with her through the maze of feelings and treatments with a sense of simply conversing with a good friend. Combining one's personal story, psychological insights, and theology into a readable text is no easy task. Beverly Sinke has done this."

Sr. Mary Lea Schneider, OSF
President, Cardinal Stritch University
Milwaukee, WI


"This remarkable book is a powerful gift to anyone who strives to be present to 'the suffering that comes.' It is a gift especially to those of us who are cancer survivors."

Jane Schaberg
Professor of Religious Studies and Women's Studies
University of Detroit Mercy


"The basic questions that nag anyone facing suffering and loss are those that have neither easy nor satisfying answers. Dr. Sinke doesn't flinch from the questions (they may indeed be yours too) which may be the reason why the reader will find the story of her journey personally profitable."

Sr. Donna Hart, IHM
Livonia, MI

# Of Related Interest...

## Cancer and Faith
*Reflections on Living with a Terminal Illness*
John Carmody

Contains over forty inspiring and comforting reflections for the terminally ill as they deal with the reality of their illness and ponder their future.

0-89622-594-1, 160 pp, $9.95

## Growing Through Pain and Suffering
Cornelius van der Poel

Using Erik Erikson's eight stages of development, this book examines why people respond to pain in certain ways and demonstrates how to accept the existence of pain and suffering in a way that encourages growth and spiritual maturity.

0-89622-636-0, 128 pp, $9.95

## Psalms for Times of Trouble
John Carmody

Openly realistic prayers, forged in the darkness and trouble of the author's own battle with terminal cancer. Inspires hope of the eternal kindness and mercy of God. Makes a thoughtful, hope-filled gift for people in pain or sorrow.

0-89622-614-X, 176 pp, $9.95

## The Pummeled Heart
*Finding Peace Through Pain*
Antoinette Bosco

This touching and amazing story of one woman's struggle to confront many forms of suffering offers a model of trust and hope in God, and gives strength to overcome evil. Readers will want to share this book with others.

0-89622-584-4, 140 pp, $7.95. Also available in cloth: 0-89622-595-X, $14.95

*Available at religious bookstores or from:*

# TWENTY-THIRD PUBLICATIONS
PO BOX 180 · 185 WILLOW STREET (◉) MYSTIC, CT 06355 · 1-800-321-0411
FAX: 1-800-572-0788  BAYARD  E-MAIL: ttpubs@aol.com
### Call for a free catalog